THE SCIENCE OF PERFECT WEIGHT

LIFESUCCESS PUBLISHING, LLC
8900 E Pinnacle Peak Road, Suite D240
Scottsdale, AZ 85255
Telephone: 800.473.7134
Fax: 480.661.1014
E-mail: admin@lifesuccesspublishing.com

ISBN: 978-1-59930-172-3
Cover : Fiona Dempsey & LifeSuccess Publishing, LLC
Layout: Fiona Dempsey & LifeSuccess Publishing, LLC

THE SCIENCE OF PERFECT WEIGHT

A NEW WAY OF THINKING, EATING AND LIVING TO ACHIEVE YOUR PERFECT WEIGHT

BOB PROCTOR &
MELONIE DODARO

Table of Contents

The information and guidance provided in this book are not intended to be a substitute for medical advice. The reader should first consult his/her health care practitioner before commencing a new exercise or implementing any suggestions regarding diet, including supplements or herbal or nutritional treatments. The author and publisher expressly disclaim responsibility for any adverse effects arising directly or indirectly from information contained in this book.

Dedication

THIS BOOK IS dedicated to all of you who believe that your goal of achieving your Perfect Weight is attainable. This book is also dedicated to all of you who believe that your goal of achieving your Perfect Weight is not attainable as this is the book that will change your mind.

Foreword

THROUGHOUT TIME, THE human race has been in pursuit of achievements that seem to drastically change and evolve as each era passes. One thing, however, has been ingrained in our mind as though it were part of our genetic make-up; maximizing our health, improving our looks and attaining our ideal weight. My friends Bob and Melonie have evolved the concept of good health and reaching your ideal weight to an exciting new level with their inspiring book, The Science of Perfect Weight.

By breaking loose from the common mindset held in today's society that every cure is just a pill away, they will transport you from where you are to where you desire to be in the most important aspect of your life - your wellness. They will guide you to this higher state of being by immersing you in the true fountain of youth. In this book they will lead you directly to your own goal of improved health and Perfect Weight. You now have in your hands the strategy that will truly work for YOU!

It brings me great honor to say that they have been my friends for a very long time and that I continue to witness their encouraging example of radiant health, happiness, vitality, and healthy weight. You will find the material in this book easy to read, remember, and so easy to do that you will walk away with lifelong results. You will want share this secret with your family and friends. Congratulations in advance on achieving your Perfect Weight.

- ***Mark Victor Hansen***

Acknowledgements

SIOBHAN SHAW HAS been an enormous help in the editing and preparation of this book and the Perfect Weight Program. With a B.A. in Psychology, a background in writing as well as the health and wellness industry, she has reviewed and contributed to the content of this book more than any other person.

MICHALE HARTTE, BASc Nutrition, RNCP, CFT, earned her Degree in Applied Nutrition. She is a Registered Nutritional Consultant Practitioner and Fitness Trainer. She designed The Perfect Weight Nutrition Plan just for you. She created a plan that you can easily integrate into your lifestyle with a few simple modifications. Michale has 14 years of experience in numerous areas of health and fitness. Her special interest is in weight loss, children's health, pre-natal, and postnatal care. She is a strong believer in preventative nutrition, which she draws on all her knowledge and experiences as a nutritional counselor, personal trainer, writer, and educator to truly get results.

CHAPTER ONE

The First Step to Change

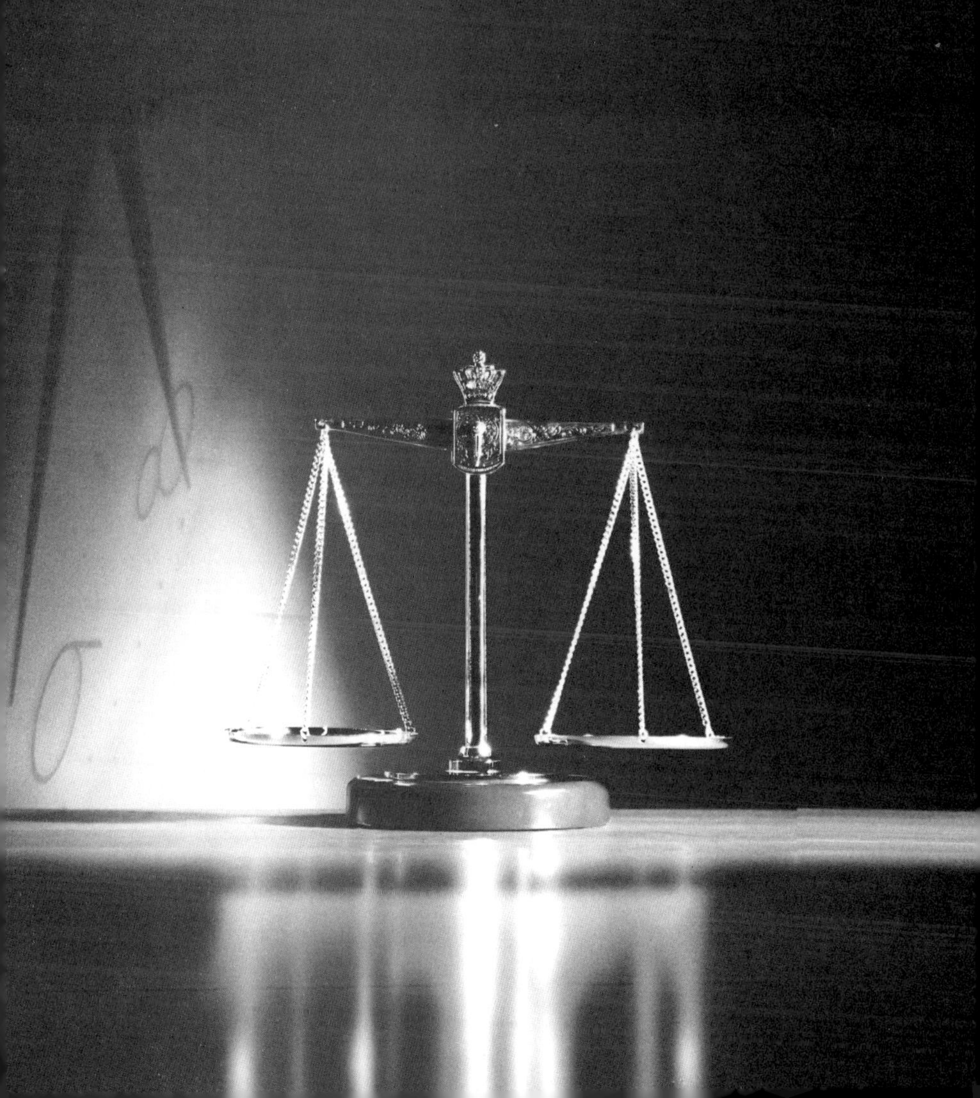

CHAPTER ONE
The First Step to Change

Instead of giving myself reasons why I can't,
I give myself reasons why I can.

– Unknown Author

Autobiography in Five Short Chapters
By Portia Nelson

I. I walk down the street.
There is a deep hole in the sidewalk.
I fall in. I am lost ... I am helpless.
It isn't my fault. It takes forever to find a way out.

II. I walk down the same street.
There is a deep hole in the sidewalk.
I pretend I don't see it. I fall in again.
I can't believe I am in the same place.
But it isn't my fault. It still takes a long time to get out.

III. I walk down the same street.
There is a deep hole in the sidewalk.
I see it there.
I still fall in ... it's a habit.
My eyes are open. I know where I am.
It is my fault. I get out immediately.

IV. I walk down the same street.
There is a deep hole in the sidewalk.
I walk around it.

V. I walk down another street.

Imagine this street. It is a beautiful picturesque street, lined with gorgeous flowering trees whose canopy surrounds you like a warm sweater. Their scent wafts down around you. The sun is streaming down, warming the pavement under your feet. The breeze is light and soothing. Homes along this street are welcoming. Children are playing and laughing. People you see are smiling and happy. They wave to you. You are standing at one end of the street. At the other end is your Perfect Weight. You know it's there — you can see it and it seems like an easy stroll down the street toward it — so you lead off. One foot in front of the other ... how difficult can it be, you wonder, to reach the end of the street and your Perfect Weight?

It's a clear path. No worries. One step, then another and another ... you stumble on a stone ... another step ... a car backs out of a driveway and doesn't see you. You stop short. Carry on. My Perfect Weight is just over there — easy to get to, you say to yourself. You move forward. There's a sidewalk café … how tempting the aroma coming from inside. A hot creamy cappuccino and a warm pastry would be nice. You sit down. Relax. Enjoy.

It's time to get up now. You linger. It's hard to leave the comfort of the café. In walk Bob Proctor and Melonie Dodaro. They know the path to your Perfect Weight. They hold out their hands. Follow them, don't look back. They will guide you past the potholes and obstacles along the street and give you the key to unlock the box that holds your Perfect Weight.

You have very likely walked down that street and fallen in the same hole that Portia Nelson refers to in her poem at the opening of this chapter — and you've probably done it more than once. We all have. The secret is to figure out why you have. If you have a weight problem, money problem, relationship problem, or business problem, understand this: all problems originate inside, not outside. They originate in the nonphysical world — they merely manifest in the material world. The Perfect Weight Program deals with paradigms; it deals with the primary cause of problems. Although this Perfect Weight Program deals specifically with weight, to your delight, you will become aware that the philosophy that is the foundation of this program — a philosophy that, by the way, you will fall in love with — can be used to accomplish any goal in your life, from wealth to Perfect Weight.

– Bob Proctor

Welcome. I am so happy and grateful to introduce you to your Perfect Weight. I am Melonie Dodaro, co-founder of the Perfect Weight Program. Bob Proctor, world-renowned motivational speaker and contributor to the bestselling DVD and book, *The Secret,* has joined forces with me to bring you closer to your Perfect Weight by introducing you to the missing piece that has eluded many of us and kept us from achieving our ideal weight.

Have you found yourself wondering why you haven't accomplished the things you desire in your life? For instance, how often have you have tried to reduce your weight? I have been in the weight-loss industry for over a decade, owned several weight-loss centers, and worked with thousands of clients. During that time have I noticed that the clients who had positive attitudes and believed that they would achieve success were always successful at achieving their goal weight. The others — the clients who made excuses for why they gained weight and had negative thoughts (whether they realized it or not) throughout their programs — rarely achieved their desired goals. You can't imagine the comments I have heard. Usually these statements begin with "I can't": *I can't eat breakfast; I can't live without my coffee; I can't get up at 6 a.m. to go running; I can't feed my family this way; I can't seem to lose weight!* You name it… I have heard them all.

When you hold the image of what you want on the screen of your mind, you are vibrating in harmony with every particle of energy that is necessary for the manifestation of your image on the physical plane. By holding that image, the people, things,

conditions, and circumstances you require are moving toward you and you toward them — because that is the law.

– Bob Proctor

After watching *The Secret,* I was inspired by its premise and began studying with the teachers from the DVD. I went to a training seminar where Bob Proctor, one of the teachers from *The Secret,* was speaking. He talked about how we attract into our lives whatever we give our attention to, whatever we focus on — good or bad. We are made up of energy and energy sends out vibrations. These vibrations are either negative or positive and you easily know what vibrations you are sending out based on how you are feeling. Think about it — when you are going on a vacation, you are excited to go. You feel free from all the daily stresses and you get very relaxed very quickly. This is a positive state of mind.

Then there are the days you wake up on the wrong side of the bed. You're out of milk. The dog has left you a little reminder that you didn't walk him last night. Traffic is a nightmare — where did all these cars come from? You are running late for work. You spill coffee on your shirt when someone cuts you off. You get to work and your boss wants to see the project you were supposed to finish, and — oh, no! — it's on your kitchen table at home! Then to top it all off in walks the customer from your worst nightmare. Nothing is going right. You wonder, why me? What did I do to deserve such a rotten day? Let me tell you.

All morning you have been cursing everyone else, feeling sorry for yourself and screaming inside "let me off this circus ride." It's likely that you woke up worrying about your day and have been running various negative thoughts through your mind without even realizing it. Those are negative vibrations. Who today has had a negative thought drift into his or her mind? When you have negative thoughts, you create negative vibrations. Those vibrations, either positive or negative, cause all of the results you are receiving and have received in the past.

Once I truly understood this and began to relate these theories to my reality, I realized that ***what was missing in the weight-loss business was the power of the mind.*** That explained why some people were successful and some were not. Just eliminate the words don't, won't, can't, shouldn't, not, and no from your vocabulary and watch what happens. You will quickly find you can do anything.

Start thinking about what you do want.

Stop thinking about what you don't want. Start thinking about what you do want. Stop avoiding change. Start listening to yourself and to the excuses you use to keep from moving forward toward your dreams and aspirations. You may say things such as "I'm too busy to … I'd love to but … If I were slimmer I'd …" You have to set your mind to your chosen goal and visualize it as though it is already yours — then watch as your dreams come true. It worked for me. I walked right up to Bob Proctor and told him I had an idea — I wanted to create a program with him to help people achieve their Perfect Weight, focusing most of the attention on the mind. He agreed, and today I am an author and the president and co-founder of LifeSuccess Perfect Weight. I tell you this because this is a perfect example of how the Law of Attraction works. When you really believe in something or really want something, you can have it. The only one who has prevented you in the past is you — your own mind. We are going to teach you how to control your mind so that you can control your results in life.

Start your journey today toward your Perfect Weight goal. Whatever it is, it can be done. When your thoughts turn negative, turn them around. Believe in yourself and your goal and follow the steps outlined in this book.

It is no secret that we, as a society, are obsessed with diet and weight. Proof of this can be seen every day in the media with the promotions of the latest fad diets featuring slim role models from Hollywood and Madison Avenue. You would think we would all be fabulously healthy and living life at our Perfect Weight without a care in the world. However, in a horribly warped contradiction, studies show that U.S. obesity rates have reached epic proportions. What is going on? Everyone you meet claims to be concerned about health and weight, but few seem to make positive changes. Why? Working in the health and wellness arena for the last decade, I've seen this problem reach frightening levels. As I have said before, I've come to the conclusion that achieving your Perfect Weight is not really about eating healthy or exercising, though they are both components to a healthy lifestyle. ***The true key to achieving your Perfect Weight is in the mind.*** It is in how we think about ourselves. It is in the lies we create and the excuses we give. It is also within our power to change and it's becoming more urgent that we do so with each passing day.

THE CURRENT STATISTICS ARE QUITE GRIM:

- Results from the 2003-2004 National Health and Nutrition Examination Survey estimate that 66% of American adults are categorized as either overweight or obese.
- One-third of children and teens between the ages of 2 and 19 are overweight or at risk of becoming so. This has nearly tripled since the 1970s.
- Nearly 78% of Americans are not meeting basic activity level recommendations.
- Approximately 25% of Americans live completely sedentary lives.
- Since 1990, there has been a 76% increase in Type II diabetes in adults 30-40 years old.
- About 300,000 deaths are attributed to obesity each year.
- In 2000, the economic cost of obesity in the United States was $117 billion.

THE AMERICAN AND CANADIAN governments, faced with the distressing reality that two-thirds of all Americans and half of all Canadians are overweight or obese, have redesigned their food pyramids, hoping to encourage people to eat healthier. Up until recently, the food guides placed emphasis on cereals, breads, and other grains; fruits and vegetables; dairy and meats; and fats and oils. The new pyramids recognize that one size does not fit all, and say you should "make smart choices from every food group ... and get the most nutrition out of your calories" (mypramid.gov). In other words, it is best to emphasize "smart choices" such as whole grains, fruit and vegetables, nuts and seeds, and healthy fats, while reducing the intake of sugar, alcohol, red meat, dairy, starchy vegetables, white pasta, and white bread — the foods that often cause weight gain and digestive problems.

How do we stop this ridiculous spiral of poor health and obesity? How do we as a collective consciousness end the madness and stop killing ourselves with the effects of processed food and sedentary lifestyles? What ever happened to survival of the fittest? If our ancestors had eaten as we do today, many of us wouldn't be here. Studies suggest that for the first time in history, American children's life expectancies are now less than those of their parents. That is not because our medical system is worse but because of what we feed our children. This is a scary statistic and one that should wake us all up. Stop bringing processed foods into your home! Get your kids moving — and that doesn't mean they should just use their video-gaming muscles! Don't go to fast-food restaurants that don't offer you wholesome, healthy options! We the people can make a difference. We just need to change our behaviors and — most important of all — our attitudes and mindset. *The Science of Perfect Weight* is about how you can create a new mindset that will create the lifestyle changes you must make to be healthy.

THE EFFECTS OF DENIAL

THE FIRST STEP IS to move past denial. For many people denial is a constant companion — so much so that they don't realize they are participating in it. Don't believe me? Let's take a quick test.

Only you – have the power to create your life.

Most people who you meet in the course of your daily life will, when asked, tell you that they are "fine." How are you? Fine. How is your family? Fine. How is your job? Fine. In reality, most of us can think of many aspects of our lives we would like to change. Perhaps we are dissatisfied with our jobs, co-workers, or bosses. Maybe our family life is either stressful, in chaos, or achingly lonely. Each person who has ever walked the planet has experienced the frustration of wanting to be more, do more, and to have a calm, balanced life. Yet most of us float through life never being consciously aware of what we do or why — and that includes the way we eat. Americans spend many billions of dollars each year on magic diet books or programs that promise to transform their lives into what they dream about, believing that these easy fixes will solve all their problems. But I want you to understand there is no magic pill. No amount of money, no person, no medical procedure, and no program will ever bring you total happiness.

The reason that none of these external sources will make your life better is that you, and only you, have the power to change the course of your life. You determine how you live, how you respond to life, and how much abundance you will experience. The power to choose your life and the ability to change anything that you don't like lies totally within you.

You may be thinking, "If this is true, then why do I feel so trapped? I don't believe that I'd ever choose to be overweight." This is a completely normal reaction. The only way to understand how to improve your life is to look within. It's a challenge to understand why you think and act the way you do. By reading this book, you have chosen to undertake that challenge, and recognize who you are and how you have created your current life. The first step in changing yourself is awareness. You must understand where you are right now and how you got there. Only then can you create something better.

Denial, according to Wikipedia, "is a defense mechanism in which a person is faced with a fact that is too painful to accept and rejects it instead, insisting that it is not true despite what may be overwhelming evidence. The subject may deny the reality of the unpleasant fact altogether (simple denial), admit the fact but deny its seriousness (minimization), or admit both the fact and seriousness but deny responsibility (transference). The concept of denial is particularly important to the study of addiction."

Food, like tobacco and alcohol, can become an addiction. We've all heard someone say, "I need chocolate!" or "You can't watch hockey without pizza and beer!" We all know young children who see candy in a colorful wrapper and will kick and scream until they get it. These people are in denial.

Denial can be deadly for some people. For instance, the signs of a heart attack are so varied and complex that they are often ignored and shrugged off as heartburn. I know of a young, vigorous firefighter trained in first aid and rescue who felt chest pains at the station one day. Instead of informing his colleagues, he carried on to the end of his shift. Driving home, he finally admitted to himself that he was in so much pain that he ought to stop at the hospital. He was lucky he did; it turned out that his "indigestion" was a heart attack. He could easily have collapsed and died during a rescue or by crashing his car, and left behind a wife and two children, all because he denied his symptoms. Denial can kill us.

We know that what we put into our bodies can eventually lead to such illnesses as diabetes, heart disease, and cancer. So why do we continue to eat processed foods, trans-fat, and refined sugars? We are living in a state of denial. It won't happen to me. The effects of denial are not easily measured, seen, or even felt for years, sometimes decades, but a life of excess eventually catches up to everyone.

HERE ARE EXAMPLES of the levels of denial–simple denial, minimization and transference–as they relate to weight.

1. SIMPLE DENIAL – IGNORING THE FACTS ALTOGETHER.

   This is the person who has diabetes and high blood pressure, takes all kinds of medications, and yet continues to eat sugary cereals and chocolate bars.

2. MINIMIZATION – ACKNOWLEDGE THE TRUTH BUT DENY ITS SERIOUSNESS.

This is the person who tells everyone that the doctor has instructed him or her to reduce weight yet continues to chow down on cheeseburgers and fries.

3. TRANSFERENCE: ACKNOWLEDGING THE FACTS AND THE SERIOUSNESS BUT DENYING RESPONSIBILITY.

   This is the person who says, "I know I'm fat, I have diabetes, and it can kill me, but my family won't change how they eat and it's too much trouble to make separate meals for myself. I can't change."

Pay attention to your denials. Think about this. Notice what you are thinking, doing, and saying. You might be saying, "I am not in denial about anything!" — which is a denial in itself. Your denial may be as simple as, "a piece of that pecan pie before bed won't hurt," or it could be as complex as, "Sure, I'm a happy enough person." If you become aware that you deny things, people, or events in your life, don't panic. I have good news: **You have the power within you to change.**

YOUR TRUE SELF

WHEN YOU COME HOME at the end of the day and are alone, who are you? Your true self is who you are when no one is looking, when no one is judging, and when you can live as you please and eat what you want. Indeed, everyone has a public and a private self. There is the person we show to the world, and the person who only we know. Often these two selves are very different. When you are at work or going about your daily life, you may consciously alter your behavior to match the person who you want other people to see. For example, maybe you order a salad for lunch with co-workers, but then scarf down a burger and fries in the car on your way home. We all do this to some extent, but if your public food self and your private food self are very different, this duality can be costly from a health perspective. Portraying an inauthentic version of who you are to the world can cost you in terms of stress, energy, honesty, and self-worth.

Furthermore, our self-worth is tied very closely to our inner self.

You may be afraid to let others see the real you for fear of being criticized or feeling embarrassed. The problem is that your self-image takes a hit every time you escape into denial because what you project conflicts with your true idea of your inner self. For example, the way you dress and the things you have around you are all a projection of who you believe yourself to be. A good example would be people who wear nothing but black, thinking that doing so will hide their weight. Who does this really fool? Or how about someone who sits in the doctor's office complaining of sore knees and, when told that the solution is simply to reduce weight, ignores the truth and asks for painkillers? The truth hurts. It's easier to pop a pill than to reduce a few pounds; denial is the path of least resistance. The reality is that you and you alone have created your present situation. No amount of covering up will change that. You cannot hide from who and what you really are.

Our self-worth is tied very closely to our inner self. Self-worth can be described as a personal judgment of worthiness that is expressed in the attitudes we hold about ourselves. The picture we hold of ourselves in our own minds is intimately connected to the value we place on ourselves. A healthy self-worth means having a positive, constructive view of yourself and your abilities. It allows you to work toward your goals and engage in rewarding relationships. An unhealthy self-worth means having a negative, pessimistic, or disapproving view of yourself, unable to see beyond limitations and problems. People with an unhealthy self-worth believe that they can't reach goals or have meaningful relationships. Often people's self-worth is directly reflected in their weight and overall health. Self-destructive behavior, such as gaining weight or smoking, reveals a negative self-image.

You can change your self-worth. This takes more effort than just chanting a few positive phrases and receiving passing approval from others. It goes much deeper. Although positive thinking and affirmations are essential, improvement also involves taking action. ***In order to truly BE great, you must first think it, then believe it, and then set goals to make it happen.***

For example, let's say that one day you are feeling a bit down because you have gained a few pounds. Then a good friend comes along and compliments you on your appearance. This makes you feel good — temporarily. The emotion is fleeting because you know you have gained weight and have done nothing to earn or "deserve" that praise. You don't feel worthy and therefore you refuse to accept it.

Now let's assume that you have started a new workout regime and have lost 4 pounds in the last week. When this same friend compliments you, you feel good, and the emotion lasts. The difference is that you took action and therefore feel worthy of the praise. When you take steps to improve yourself, you automatically improve the image you hold of yourself in your mind, which in turn affects the attitude you project. Self-worth has less to do with feeling good than it does with feeling right. Make no mistake; there is a substantial difference between the two. This feeling of right has nothing to do with right versus wrong. It's about feeling genuine and authentic inside.

You may be thinking that you haven't felt right in a very long time. You haven't felt good about yourself or your overall health. You know you should skip the doughnut and coffee this morning, but you're in a hurry and it's easy. Lunch should include vegetables or fruit, but the hot dog is quick. In fact, it may have been months since you actually had fresh, green vegetables. Our stressful lives convince us that we're doing the best we can — but are we? Each day we make small choices that together form the landscape of our lives.

When we are forced to perform under stress, whether that stress is a ticking clock, traffic accident, or screaming child, our true nature shows itself very clearly. Our ingrained habits and belief systems (paradigms) take over, and we live on autopilot, no matter what we say we really want. Thus, denial becomes our constant companion, alleviating the guilt and burying the true causes of our unhealthy lifestyle.

So why not just go on a diet and get in shape? According to a recent dieting survey of 500 adults by Health/Insight Express, 25% of people who have tried to reduce weight have done so using at least 20 different diets, and 60% of all dieters have regained those pounds they once lost. The survey noted that when dieters get tired of the routine of less food and more exercise, they tend to gain back all those pounds they lost, and then some.

This is true and has been true for decades, but if it is really so, why do some people reduce literally hundreds of pounds and keep it off while others don't? The difference lies in the mind. Successful dieters changed their mindsets and believed they could achieve their goals. The problem with most people who struggle with their weight is that they view weight as a temporary issue to be fixed rather than a lifestyle to be lived. Thus, they look for quick solutions such as harmful fad diets. They don't make the effort to establish healthy eating habits that they can maintain long-term.

Few people ever take the time to develop a true plan for a healthy life. Most of the people you see each day are living on autopilot, doing exactly the same things they did the day before, learning nothing new, and experiencing the same results. They are doing time in a prison of their own making; unaware of the life they are missing.

IF YOU BELIEVE YOU CAN OR CAN'T YOU ARE RIGHT! What are you going to decide to believe right now?

PROCRASTINATION CAN BE a big obstacle in attaining your Perfect Weight. Many people put off diet changes saying, "I'll start tomorrow, or next Monday, or on New Year's Day." They tell themselves they are too busy right now to focus, and they'll get to it later. They might go so far as to commit to going to the gym and even buy a membership, but they never go.

"Put off today what you can do tomorrow" is the procrastinator's motto. Procrastination is a sort of paralysis. You may look at other people being productive and feel like you have a ton of bricks on your lap and can't move. The indecision and sheer inertia can play havoc on your plans to reach your goals.

Contrary to how it may feel sometimes, we all have the same amount of time in any given day — no more, no less. Time does not discriminate. Without a commitment of time, you will not change your health habits and you will not reach your goal of attaining your Perfect Weight. You will continue to stumble through your life accepting your behavior rather than creating what you desire.

You make an unconscious choice to procrastinate. Now make a conscious choice to get out of your own way. You are the cause and the effect. Become accountable for your inaction. Design yourself a chart, and on that chart put a gold star for every time you reach the end of your day having made good food choices and exercised, per your day's plan. Place a red "X" on the chart every time you slip. Set a certain number of Xs that you cannot go past, say five in a month. If you have five or fewer Xs at the end of the month, then treat yourself to some special reward — not food related.

Another good way to get things done quickly and efficiently is to learn to say NO to people and situations that may not be important but can take you off track. For instance, perhaps you are all set to exercise when your best friend phones asking you to go to a movie instead. Many people would use the invitation as an excuse to get out of exercising. This may help your social life but it won't help your waistline.

A great way to deal with procrastination is to use the KISS strategy: Keep it simple, silly. Let's say you are indecisive about what to eat everyday or what exercise to do. Peel off all the layers and go with the easiest solution. Walk around the block. Eat chicken and salad. You don't need to make an elaborate dinner or plan to become a gold-medal athlete overnight. You just need to do something every day to move closer to your Perfect Weight.

For a moment, set aside your fears of what others think, what happened in the past, and what you have to do tomorrow. Let it go and focus on this one thing: What would your life be like if you reached your Perfect Weight? How would your life change? What would you accomplish for yourself and for your family? What greatness would come to you, and how would your confidence and belief in yourself be affected? Focus on that idea and let go of anything holding you back.

Few people expect greatness. Few expect abundance. Few expect happiness. But you can make a choice to expect great things. Often people focus on scarcity, not plenty. Or they focus on failure, not success. Achieving a new and healthy life will not be easy at first, but it will be one of the most rewarding gifts you ever give yourself. Today is your chance to focus and look for what is rightfully yours. You deserve to have and be anything your mind can create in all areas of your life. Now let's begin with achieving your Perfect Weight.

PERFECT WEIGHT

SO WHAT IS YOUR Perfect Weight? There are numerous charts and measures that tell you what the suggested weight should be for your height, gender, and age. Ignore all of those. Your Perfect Weight is about how you feel physically and emotionally. It is whatever you want it to be. It's about how you interact with other people, what makes you feel great in your clothes, the right dress size for you, how much energy you need to get through your day, whether or not your knees hurt, or whether you are healthy. You may need to shed pounds or put them on. You may simply want to feel healthier, or be able to walk up a flight of stairs without getting winded. You may just want to be able to zip up your pants without sucking in your stomach and then having it roll out over your waistline. Whatever it is for you — what it is that makes you feel confident, self-assured, sexy, healthy, strong, vibrant, and free — that's your Perfect Weight.

Weight is not something to be cured; it is something to be managed. Individuals who have achieved their Perfect Weight are not lucky or superhuman, even though they may seem that way to you at this moment. They have consciously or unconsciously made a decision to be healthy.

You may remember the old adage, "Early to bed, early to rise, makes a man healthy, wealthy, and wise." This time-honored saying can be interpreted to mean it is your will that creates your destiny. When I hear this saying I picture people who go to bed early, eat well, exercise, listen to their bodies, and are kind to themselves, and for that they are rewarded with health, wealth, and wisdom. They know what it takes to reach their goals. **They don't foolishly stand by and let life manage them; they manage their life.** To be at your Perfect Weight you must make the decision to do what is necessary to move you in the direction of your goal.

It is your Perfect Weight, no one else's. I encourage you to never step on a scale again. Do not waste time weighing yourself. Do not focus on the number; that is actually a detriment to releasing weight. When you focus on the number, your sub-conscious focuses on it, too. Every time you step on the scale, your mind will fixate on how many pounds you've lost. Unfortunately, your sub-conscious will try to "help" by finding them again. Instead of focusing on these lost pounds, picture yourself at your Perfect Weight. Gauge your success with how you feel, the compliments you receive, the milestones you pass, the changes in your overall fitness and health, and how well your clothing fits. Good health is not about achieving a perfect number; it is about improving your life. The changes in what you eat and the way you do things will affect your overall weight, but this isn't a race or competition. It's a lifestyle change. If you do want to chart your progress then I suggest measuring yourself in a few key areas such as your chest, waist, hips, and thighs.

The belief that you can change is the key. Believing you can change encourages commitment to the process and enhances the likelihood of success. Only you can know your exact circumstances, and only you can find the solution, but if you don't believe there is a solution in the first place you will never find it. Stopping and searching for solutions takes time and effort. Many people are so convinced that they will fail that they are not willing to even try to change. For example, you might believe that you are so overweight that only a miracle will help you at this point, so you don't even try. No answer ever revealed itself to one who was not searching. So listen up, all you couch potatoes: you need to get off the couch, create a plan, stick to it, and remember that the one thing you can know for certain is that another day of watching TV will not help you achieve your Perfect Weight. No one has ever lost weight sitting in front of the TV snacking on chips and popcorn. It's time to do something. NO MORE EXCUSES!

This is not to say that change is easy. People do not change their lives with a snap of their fingers. Although your awareness of your capabilities and the reality that you are currently living may change in an instant, the circumstances and relationships in your life usually take more effort. However, these repeated efforts are critical to bringing about lasting change.

THERE ARE REALLY only two basic reasons that people change:

1. Circumstances make them change.
2. They choose to change.

WE SEE THE truth in these two statements every day in our lives. Let's consider the first one. Have you ever gone to the doctor and been told you must reduce weight or suffer dire health consequences? Have you ever experienced a time when you needed your body to perform — maybe you were forced to walk a long distance or climb a long set of stairs — and found that you just couldn't do it? Change for many people only occurs as a result of distress. If you choose to see these events for what they are, and don't attach your self-worth or emotions to them, they can be catalysts for positive changes. If a doctor warns you that you have to reduce weight or risk serious illness or even death, let that be the catalyst to a new lifestyle. If you're frightened by the fact that you couldn't climb a few flights of stairs in an emergency, let that be a reminder of the importance of being fit. Whatever you do, don't view these events as an indictment of who you are as a person; the results can be devastating. Distressful events will happen in your life, but your reaction to those events determines the outcome. Those reactions are 100% your choice.

Now let's take a look at the second possibility — that we choose to change. How many times do you see a diet guru on TV and feel guilty that you are sitting on the couch with a bag of cookies? Or perhaps a friend or family member offered to work out with you and you found some excuse not to? Have you nagged yourself about reducing weight and promised to start next Monday? Does all that guilt and nagging mean that you will change? No. You will only change the way you do things by choice — when you truly want to change and are ready to do so. You will never be nagged, pressured, or pushed by someone else into lasting change.

You must decide that you want to change. Not next week or next year — RIGHT NOW! Urgency is a key component to making serious and lasting changes, and the decision to change is necessary. Why? Because people are more likely to act on — and stick to — their own decisions rather than someone else's. You must decide for yourself that you want to change, not because your children, spouse, or parents say you should. Not because your doctor or fitness coach says it's the right thing to do. Not because some "expert" says so. You must decide to change to a healthy lifestyle because you want to and because you have made the choice to do so.

THE POWER OF YOU

We become what we think about. Thinking is the highest function of which we are capable and we think in images. The importance of this point cannot be stressed too much, as it will prove to be critical to your success in this program. The images you hold in your mind ultimately control your behavior, which in turn, controls your results. To alter the images that control your mind you must begin by altering the way you think. This will become more and more obvious as you work your way through this program.

- Bob Proctor

THE IDEA THAT we create our own reality is downright painful for many, or at least distasteful. Many people honestly believe that they have no choices, and even those who do believe they can choose often beat themselves up for past choices they've made — diet failures, lack of fitness — the results of which they are living now.

We are totally responsible for whatever manifests in our lives — all of it. This again begs the question, why would we create bodies that are overweight, fatigued, stressed out, and not physically fit? Why would we choose to do any of that to ourselves? No one creates these things deliberately, yet we've all done it at one time or another. The key to changing is to understand exactly HOW we do it. What is the process of creation, of manifestation?

Many people have heard of the Law of Attraction, which basically states that you get what you focus on. Unfortunately, many people who think they are focusing on creating their Perfect Weight are really focusing on pounds. For example, have you ever set a goal, perhaps even written it down, to achieve a certain clothing size? Did you then spend your days constantly hopping on the scale? Worrying over each pound? Continually calculating how many pounds had to disappear and in what time frame? While your goal was to achieve a certain clothing size, you spent most of your time focusing on pounds and that, therefore, is what you attracted. The reverse is also true. When you focus on what you want, whether it is a certain clothing size or your Perfect Weight, you'll manifest only that. For instance, let's say you want to be a size 8. If you think in terms of the number of pounds you need to reduce in order to reach that goal, say 20 pounds, then all your energy and thought processes will be focused on losing those 20 pounds. Your sub-conscious mind won't think in terms of losing or gaining, it only fixates on the fact that 20 pounds is the goal. If, however, you were to focus on the clothing size and imagine yourself wearing size 8 — how it feels to put on size 8 clothes, eating as a person who already wears a size 8 — then your mind will focus on becoming a size 8. The same holds true for your Perfect Weight. Let's say you want to weigh 140 pounds. The key is not to concentrate on how many fewer pounds you need to weigh to successfully attain that goal; the key is to imagine yourself as already weighing 140 pounds, thinking as you would if you were 140 pounds, exercising like a person who weighs 140 pounds, and making the food chooses a 140-pound person makes. **See it, believe it, feel it, be it. It's a simple concept, but quite out of the norm for most people.**

As we mature, we have experiences that shape who we are and what we believe. These experiences may be good or bad, but each event causes us to make a decision about what we believe, and that decision, in turn, affects how we live our lives from that point forward. The belief systems or programs set in place at a very young age affect and alter the way we see the world. For example, if you were constantly told to clean your plate, that habit may carry into adulthood. If you were encouraged and praised for good grades rather than for playing sports, you may have decided that intelligence is more important that being physically fit. If you were hurt in a relationship or lonely as a child, you may have decided that you can't trust other people and found that additional weight was a way to keep people away. These belief systems and programs that were set in place when we were children persist through our lives. They affect our attitudes and feelings toward food and overall health, which then manifest in our lives through actions and behaviors that produce the results we see in our lives.

The belief systems or programs set in place at a very young age affect and alter the way we see the world.

So you can see how events we experienced as children are carried forward as beliefs into adulthood. It has been said that 80% of what a child decides about himself is in place by the time that child is 4 years old. From the ages of 4 to 8, another 10% of that child's beliefs are constructed. By the age of 18, 95% of what we believe about ourselves has been formed and produces the perspective from which we view and make sense of our world. As we all have had different experiences, we all see the world slightly differently. This means that we don't necessarily see things as they are; we perceive them through the filter of our beliefs. Thus, we create our own version of reality.

EFFECTING CHANGE

HUMANS ARE THE only species that ponders the past and uses its lessons to change the future. However, few people stop to evaluate what they believe about themselves or why. Belief systems and habits learned from events, family, or your environment can move you forward or hold you back from successfully transforming your life. One of the first steps to change is to ask why.

Years ago, I heard a story about a woman who was baking a ham. Her daughter asked why she cut the ends off the ham prior to baking, expecting to hear some great culinary secret. Her reply was, "Because that's the way your grandmother did it." So the young girl went to her grandmother and asked the same question. Her grandmother replied, "Because that's the way my mother did it." The young girl then went to her great-grandmother, who was quite old and fragile, and asked her why she cut the ends off the ham. The old woman replied, "Because we were very poor and didn't have a baking pan large enough unless I cut the ends off."

This is a simple illustration of adopting someone else's belief systems without having all the facts. Old rules do not necessarily make sense in new environments or circumstances, yet they continue to be passed on. This is especially noticeable in people's belief systems about food. Why do you think people who are overweight all their lives tend to produce children who are also overweight? Or, why do you think that wealthy people often raise children who continue to attract wealth? Are these groups of people that different? Absolutely not; in fact, in most ways they are the same. One big difference, however, is in their mindset. Overweight people tend to focus on their inability to reduce weight, thus attracting more weight and creating belief systems within themselves that they are overweight. In other words, they think of themselves as fat, and therefore they become so. Wealthy people focus on wealth, so it seems they attain it more easily. They think wealthy. This is one reason you hear of people who were born to poverty yet became wealthy — the Oprahs of the world — who used the power of their mind to move from being dirt poor to becoming some of the wealthiest people in the country.

It isn't luck that changes such people's lives for the better; it is will and determination. It is the thoughts they think. It is knowing that they can achieve whatever they set out to accomplish. I'd be willing to venture that Oprah never doubted that she could be a success. She may not have known what form that success would take, but more than likely she had a positive outlook on life. People who are struggling financially often say they are broke. By thinking this, by accepting this circumstance, they will stay broke. If they changed their thinking to, "I am financially secure," they would much more easily become just that. You can trick your mind into thinking whatever it is you want to think. You just have to be aware of your thoughts and their context. And just as poverty can be a state of mind, so can obesity. Anyone who is morbidly obese can choose to become fit and healthy and succeed, but it must be a conscious and sincere choice. He or she must first put in place a decision to have a healthy and abundant mindset. Even if we cannot immediately change where we live, work, or play, we can immediately change our perspective of the world. By doing this, we create the desire and passion needed to aggressively pursue the healthy lives we deserve.

Watch your thoughts; they become words. Watch your words; they become actions. Watch your actions; they become habits. Watch your habits; they become character. Watch your character; it becomes your destiny.

– Frank Outlaw

NOTES

CHAPTER TWO

The New Mindset

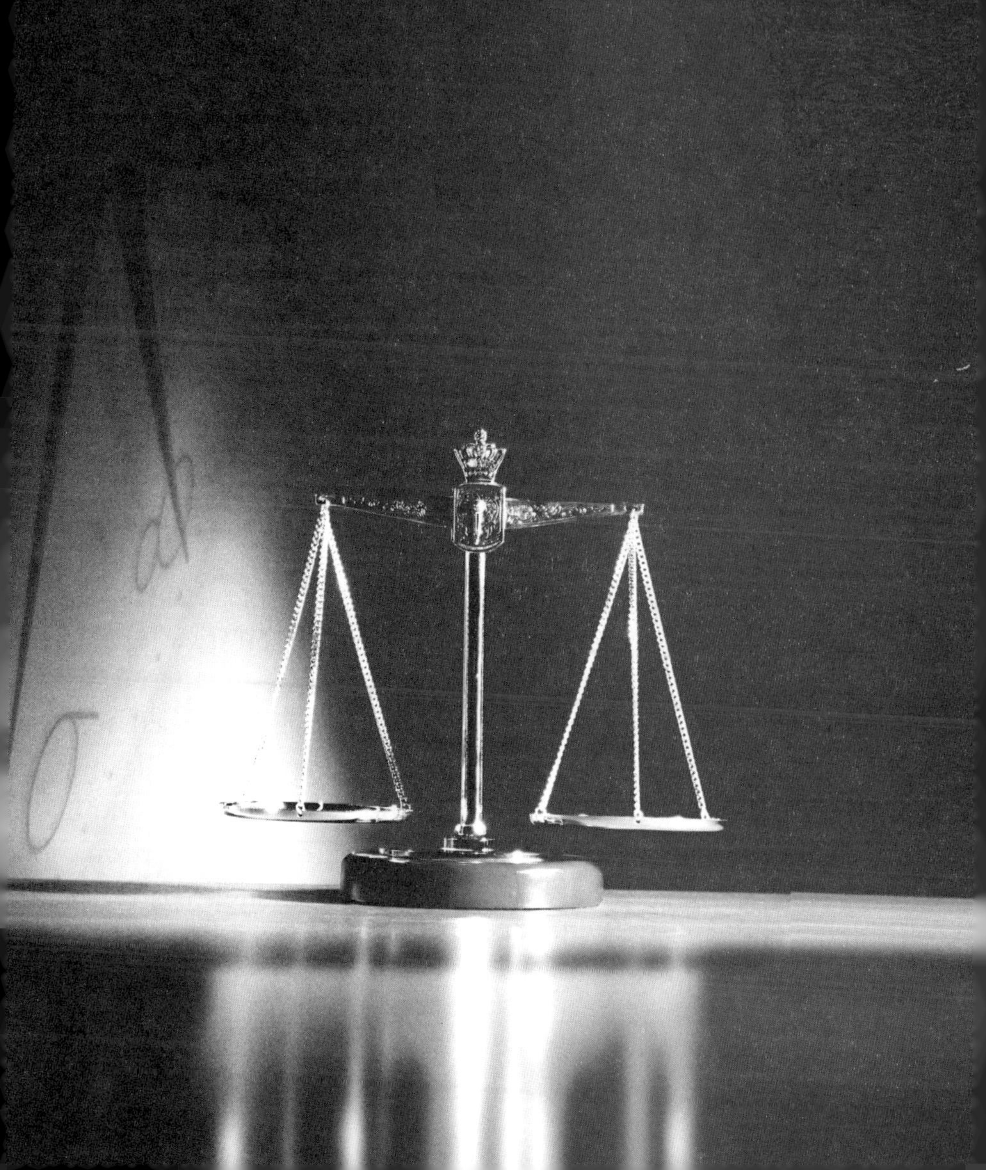

CHAPTER TWO
The New Mindset

You see, I know that you already know what you have to do to be at your Perfect Weight ... the problem is you're not doing it. The secret to success in this program is to gain an understanding of why you're not doing it, what the primary cause of the problem is and then correcting it.

– Bob Proctor

We've all heard the phrase, "You are what you eat." I completely disagree; you are what you think. What you eat is the manifestation of what you think. As we just discussed, to understand how to change your thinking about achieving your Perfect Weight, you must first understand how the mind works. The mind is an incredibly powerful tool, yet few people ever stop to think about what creates our thought patterns, feelings, and actions. Therefore, they have no idea what is responsible for how they experience their lives. The answer lies in the concept of attitude.

When we think of attitude, most people envision a type of positive thinking or having a bright and cheery demeanor. While that is an important aspect of attitude, it is only partially true. Attitude is a composite of your thoughts, feelings, and actions — not one of the three, but all of them working together in seamless combination. These thoughts, feelings, and actions are a product of our conditioned behavior, which includes how we were raised, how we've been educated, and who has influenced our lives. We are all a product of our individual experiences, and we each have a unique attitude concerning our health and fitness. To understand how these ideas and actions become ingrained in our behavior, it helps to understand how we learn.

Starting now you will learn how to take responsibility, to live in the present and not the past, to work through your fears, and to stop denying and procrastinating. Everything we know we have learned in four stages:

1. **Unconscious Incompetence.**
2. **Conscious Incompetence.**
3. **Conscious Competence.**
4. **Unconscious Competence.**

TAKE THE EXAMPLE of how a baby learns to walk. A baby first crawls to move around in the world, not knowing any other way and maybe not even knowing that there is any other way (unconscious incompetence). Eventually the baby recognizes that there's another way to move, and soon develops the desire to walk; yet still hasn't mastered the technique and has to settle for holding onto furniture and practicing (conscious incompetence). Soon the baby learns to concentrate and take a few short steps at a time without falling (conscious competence). Finally, the baby becomes so competent that he or she can walk without even having to think about it since it has become second nature (unconscious competence). Once a process is learned, the mind moves that process into the subconscious, becoming a part of us that we no longer think about. This same process is at work when we learn to ride a bicycle, drive a car, or use a computer.

Let's look at this process as it relates to weight:

1. **Unconscious Incompetence** – this can also be described as - what you don't know, you don't know. You don't know that you have not had the right diet and tools to reach your Perfect Weight.

2. **Conscious Incompetence** – or in other words what you know you don't know – you know that something is missing in the quest to reach your Perfect Weight but what it is, eludes you.

3. **Conscious Competence** – what you know you know –you know you have a weight problem and you know you have not been able to control it.

4. **Unconscious Competence** – what you don't know you know – you have the power to manage your weight. It has been with you all the time – it is your mind.

OUR MIND ALWAYS thinks in pictures. If I told you to think of your car, your home, or a cheeseburger, instantly pictures of these things would flash upon the screen of your mind. This is why we are able to drive to someone's house that we have been to before, yet can't give street names or a house number; or when taking directions we use landmarks instead of streets to guide us. If someone tells us to turn left at the gas station, we see it in our mind and automatically know where it is. If I ask you to think of your mind, you have no picture. You might get a picture of your brain, but your brain is not your mind any more than your elbow is. Your mind exists in every cell of your body. It's hard to understand your mind and how it works, unless we have a picture, so to illustrate and explain this process, we will be using the stick person example below developed in the 1930s by Dr. Thurman Fleet in San Antonio, Texas and made popular by Bob Proctor.

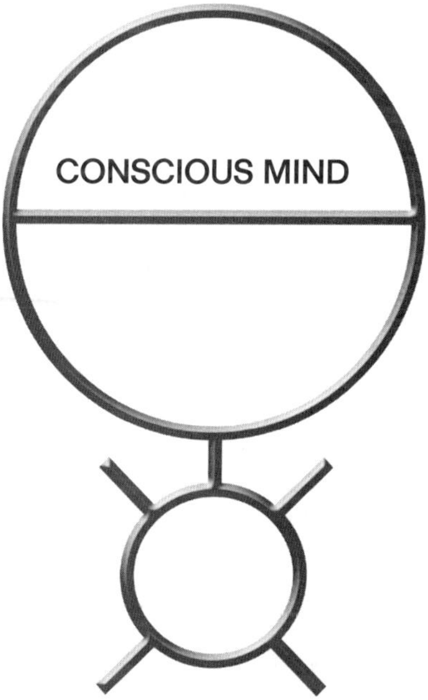

CONSCIOUS MIND

THE TOP CIRCLE represents your mind, or your thoughts, and the bottom circle represents your body, or your actions. The mind is divided into the conscious and the sub-conscious. The conscious mind is the area that receives all the input and experiences from the outside world. As you are faced with new events and ideas, your conscious mind has the ability to accept or reject any information it receives. When thoughts come to you from your surroundings, the conscious mind is the filter that allows you to choose only those ideas and events with which you want to be emotionally involved. The conscious mind is also where you create the dreams and goals that you want for your life.

It is estimated that given today's media bombardment we are exposed to tens of thousands of images per day. We can effectively capture or process approximately 1,000 of these images on a conscious level. The information age has increased the complexity of what we are exposed to in our lives. Although in many ways this makes our lives more efficient and easy, it also means that our mind must constantly choose what to process. Like most people, you probably don't think of this as an active choice, but it is. That's how it is that two people can be at the same event and yet remember two completely different versions.

If we are constantly inundated with negative messages, we are bound to choose negative thoughts and ideas that will be stored in our sub-conscious mind. We then become negative people with negative ideas and opinions — not only of the events in our lives, but also of ourselves. If we want to think, feel, and act more positively, we must guard our sub-conscious with our conscious mind by carefully choosing what ideas engage our emotions and what images we view repeatedly.

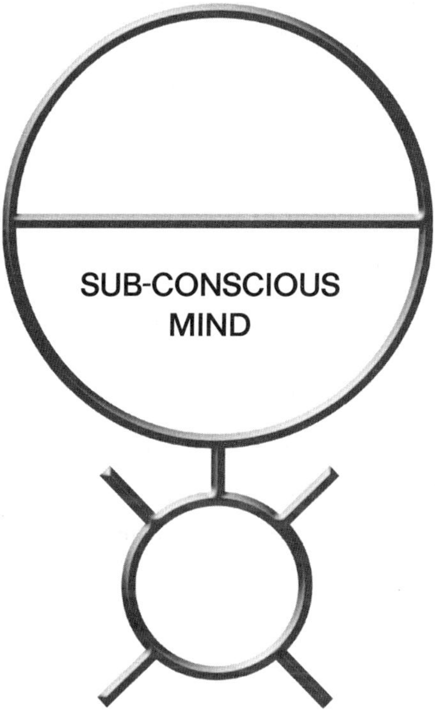

SUB-CONSCIOUS MIND

THIS IS THE "emotional mind" or "feeling mind." The ancient Greeks called it "the heart of hearts." The sub-conscious mind only has one answer to all commands it receives from the conscious mind, and that answer is "YES!" In the smash-hit DVD *The Secret,* James Arthur Ray tells us that it replies like a genie with, "Your wish is my command!"

The sub-conscious mind has no ability to accept or reject thoughts. This is why it is important to monitor thoughts and ideas as we receive them in our conscious mind. The sub-conscious mind is a blank screen, and any thoughts we accept will resurface on this screen. If we worry about something happening, then the sub-conscious mind will move us in the direction of having that negative thing happen. For example, if you say or think you are clumsy; this thought may make you trip on a crack in the sidewalk.

Likewise, if we create a positive idea of how we want events to unfold or how we want to respond to the unfortunate things that happen in our lives, then the sub-conscious mind can, and will, exhibit that positive result. Worrying and focusing on what you don't want takes just as much energy and time, if not more, than focusing on what you do want. It also works. You will always attract more of the same energy that you are in harmony with, and if it is negative, then that's what you will receive.

The encouraging message from this is that we can monitor our conscious mind. More importantly, we can teach ourselves to increase our positive results, as Napoleon Hill describes in *Think and Grow Rich*. Hill encourages us to create the thoughts and ideas that we want. By repeating those thoughts, we can manifest the realities in our lives.

THE BODY

THE BODY IS the physical form and machine that is instructed daily by our dominant thoughts and actions. The body carries out actions based on directions from the conscious

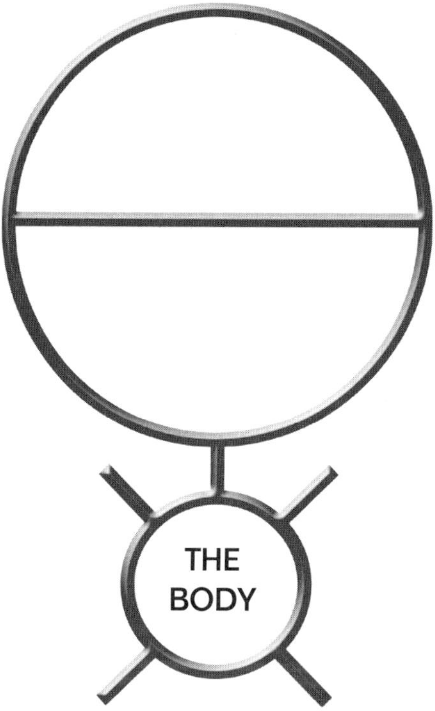

and sub-conscious mind. It is the evidence of what is held in the mind. For example, let's say you decide that you want to be a public speaker. If you are nervous and worry about saying something inappropriate, or are concerned that someone will make fun of you, then those thoughts will manifest in the body as sweaty palms, embarrassment, and stumbling over words. However, if you spend time imagining how positively your audience will respond, how articulate you will sound, and how energized you will feel, that will manifest in the body as well. You will be confident and filled with energy, and your audience can't help but respond positively to you. When we intentionally change the thoughts to which we give the most focus and energy, and repeat these thoughts until they become desires, they are impressed upon our sub-conscious mind and become emotions. Our bodies put those emotions into action and our actions become our results.

PARADIGMS

A PARADIGM, WHICH can be a habit, belief, attitude, work practice, or expectation, gives you the understanding to interpret and approach the world around you. When you examine your paradigms around weight, you may find that your present results are not the results you want. Your objective of reaching your Perfect Weight is to move your conditioned results into line with what you want. For instance, let's say that you used to drink one glass of red wine every evening, but to reach your Perfect Weight you have changed that to a glass of water with a lemon slice instead. This is a paradigm shift.

Bob Proctor, in the Perfect Weight Program, said it this way: "You see, I know that you already know what you have to do to be at your Perfect Weight; the problem is you're not doing it. The secret to success in this program is to gain an understanding of why you're not doing it, what the primary cause of the problem is, and then correcting it. Go back to a time you when you were a child in school and you did something you weren't supposed to do. When the teacher asked you, 'Why did you do that?' your probable reply was, 'I don't know.' And, then the teacher would respond, 'What do you mean, you don't know? You know you weren't supposed to do that.' And as you dropped your head, you would say, 'I know.'"

The insidious part of this is that we carry this silly, "I don't know" concept into our adult life. We do things we know we shouldn't do — things we don't want to do — and we do them anyway. We are conditioned to believe that it's our behavior that is causing the unwanted results in our life. But that's not true. We're forever attempting to change those behavior patterns: eat less, eliminate starchy foods, and exercise more often — all without success. Or, we're successful for a short period of time, but then we start going down the same street, falling in the same hole. Unfortunately, some people stay on that street for their entire life.

There are millions of people in every country in the world going on special diets to reduce weight. These people are not trying to reach their Perfect Weight; their whole obsession is with losing weight. There's a dual problem with this. First, they believe that food — eating the wrong food or eating too much food — is the cause of their problem, which is not true. Their eating habit is a secondary cause of their problem, but it's the primary cause that needs to be corrected if the results are going to permanently change. Second, when you lose anything — it doesn't matter what it is, from your car keys to those 20 pounds — you are sub-consciously programmed to immediately begin to look for it. And, unfortunately, when it comes to weight loss, you find it.

The Perfect Weight Program is going to do what Portia Nelson described in Chapter Five of the little poem at the beginning of the book: take you down another street.

The simplest and most comprehensive definition of a paradigm that we have ever come across is that it is a multitude of habits, and habits are concepts expressed in action without any conscious thought.

"To ignore the power of paradigms to influence your judgment is to put yourself at significant risk when exploring the future. To be able to shape your future you have to be ready and able to change your paradigm."

- Joel Barker

ARMED WITH PARADIGMS, you approach and react to the world around you, interpreting what you see and experience according to your shared understanding and certain culturally determined guidelines. A paradigm, in a sense, tells you that there is a game, what the game is, and how to play it successfully. A paradigm shift, then, is a change to a new game or a new set of rules. And when the rules change, the whole world will appear to change. And remember, we are going to go down a different street.

"People do not resist change, people resist being changed."

- Michael Basch

OUR HABITS

ONE WAY TO change negative beliefs you hold about yourself is by changing your habits. Do you have a habit that confirms a belief about yourself? Is that habit serving you well, or is it confirming a belief about yourself that you wish was different? For example, do you always "super-size" your meals?

If so, then this is confirming a belief that you are super-sized. You may reject the idea that this is so, but actions speak louder than words. Only by choosing and committing to a new habit will you eventually change your belief about yourself, as you create new proof based on your actions.

So how do you begin to change your beliefs and form new, more positive health habits? The first thing to do is stop lying to yourself. We all do it. How many times have you promised yourself to stick to a healthy portion size and not eat too much, and have instead gone to the fridge and eaten everything in sight?

Marc is a good example of what can happen when you lie to yourself.

My girlfriend and I made a pact to get in shape last summer. We were supposed to eat healthy lunches then meet at the gym three days a week. She did great and had a wonderful positive attitude — but I didn't. I found myself hiding the fast food wrappers and making excuses for why my weight didn't change. I cringed just thinking about the gym and, more often than not, found some excuse not to go.

It wasn't long before she achieved her goal, and I constantly belittled the achievement because I felt so angry with myself for sneaking around and doing things we'd agreed not to do. The truth is, she wanted to change and I didn't. One night, when we were supposed to have dinner with her family, she called and asked me not to go. She pointed out how I'd been acting and said she wouldn't be treated that way in front of her family. I was shocked. I didn't even realize that my insecurity and anger had caused her such pain.

Three weeks and four dozen roses later, we were at the gym every day, and I now tell everyone how proud I am of what she's accomplished. I finally made the decision to get healthy for myself, not because she wanted me to, but because I wanted to ... and that made all the difference.

BABY STEPS

CHANGING YOUR ENTIRE lifestyle may seem a little overwhelming at first, but you can ease into it by taking a few baby steps to form new healthy habits:

1. **Envision the end result.** You are not changing a habit for the sake of change itself, but because doing so will get you closer to achieving or having your Perfect Weight. If you have a habit of watching TV for a few hours every night and munching on a bag of potato chips, then turn the TV off and substitute reading or a walk.

2. **Take a reality assessment.** What's working well, what needs improvement, and what's getting in the way of your progress? Your exercise routine of lifting weights may be going perfectly well, but what if you would really like to find a more interesting way to tone your muscles? Put that on a list of things that are important to you and start working in that area.

3. **Pick a challenge – any challenge.** You don't have to pick a big challenge to start with. Think in terms of improving one percent a day – something very attainable. For example, if you drink several cups of coffee or tea a day but want to get off caffeine, start by drinking one less cup

per day or even one half cup less. Within a short time, you will have weaned yourself from the habit.

4. **Action is the key.** Form a plan for staying on track. Keep a written record of your progress. It is easy to forget the little victories, but going back and looking at a journal of success – even in the smallest areas – gives you a mental boost and encourages you to stick with your plan.

BY USING THESE baby steps — if you really commit to and persist with your new habits — I guarantee that you will have a new perspective and belief about who you are and what you can accomplish. Then you can move on to choosing the next healthy habit that you want to develop and strengthen.

People develop their beliefs about what they can or can't accomplish from even the smallest events. Words spoken by a spouse, parent, or loved one can affect your belief in your ability to change. Although family can be supportive, they also remember every failure and often point them out. You may have family or friends that constantly tell you that you are fine the way you are and just to accept it — but if you don't feel fine, then you're not. You have to decide if you will let other people limit your life.

Each one of us must remember that it is not what we are born with or without that determines who we will become. By the same token, you cannot blame others for your success or failure, as this is the road to irresponsibility and helplessness. You can only change yourself and the way you interact with others. This is the path to true happiness and success.

Knowing that you are in complete and total control of your own destiny, no matter what happens or what others say, gives you the freedom to find your true self and determine who you will become.

POOR ME

DO YOU EVER get sick of people disclaiming responsibility for their actions or lives? How many times a day do you hear people say, "It is not my fault"? How many times have you said it? A destructive paradigm that many people hold onto is the "victim syndrome." This does not mean that these people may not have experienced an unfortunate turn of events, but the event does not determine the outcome. That is determined by your reaction to that event. If you decide to face each difficulty with the attitude of "poor me," then that is exactly what you will get: a poor life. Viewing yourself as a victim of life rather than a participant weakens your resolve to create change. It is very easy to feel trapped and remain a victim for your whole life.

This "poor me" syndrome or victim mentality is stifling, and people can get caught, feeling powerless in their ability to move forward. They will constantly cry about their lot in life — I'm too fat! I have no friends! — yet they can be found sitting at home alone on the couch in front of the TV rather than doing something about it, like joining a hiking club where they could meet other people and get some exercise at the same time. You know these people. Have you ever been to dinner at a family member's house and "Cousin Sally" is sitting sulking in a chair, not participating in the conversation because she is having a bad day? Or do you know someone who is constantly blaming the cat, the car, or the boss for whatever went wrong that day? We all do it occasionally — fall into the trap of playing the victim and the blame game. No more! You need to be done with that if you truly want to achieve your dreams!

Once you become aware of the victim mentality, you will discover immediately how negative and destructive it really is. You will also find that you are not really a victim, in most circumstances, except in your own mind. You have the power to change if you want to. Many people, unfortunately, move from a victim mentality to an excuse mentality. By choosing to shift blame to something other than themselves, they don't take ownership of their own lives or health. You frequently see this if you ask people why they have given up their exercise routines or resumed bad habits. They will offer excuses rather than acknowledge that they chose to take that action — no one made them. Many people never realize that they have excused themselves right out of living and have started down a destructive path that leads to death. Alcoholics Anonymous has a saying; "There are a million excuses for picking up a drink, but no good reason." Excuses abound for not living a healthy life, but real reasons are few. Stop making excuses and choose to change for the better.

You will also find that you are not really a victim, in most circumstances.

To break the vicious cycle of excuses, half-truths, and anger you have been living with, you must first make a decision. By mastering the art of making decisions you will bring more benefit to your life than any other lesson you could study.

Mastering the ability to make effective decisions quickly will create for you what many people would consider to be a charmed life. It will also keep you in a leadership role that is envied by many and understood by few. Decision-makers go to the top, while those who do not make decisions flounder.

- Bob Proctor

DECISION MAKERS ARE the movers and shakers of the world. They are leaders and because of that become successful. How do they do that? By understanding that every decision is actually the answer to a question. Every action has an equal and opposite reaction: up – down; right – wrong; inside – outside; yes – no; cold – hot; black – white; question – answer; fat – thin. The laws of the universe hold the answer to any question; you just need to know how to tune into that frequency.

This program has, as its foundation, the natural laws of the universe; you are bringing your life into harmony with everything that is good.

- Bob Proctor

By understanding these laws and altering your life to work in harmony with them, you will find that you are able to make good decisions and reach your potential — in this case, achieving your Perfect Weight. Making a decision brings order to your existence, and order brings results. Let's say you make the decision to reach your Perfect Weight. By deciding to lay out the framework of the plan, you set yourself up for success. Simply moving forward without a plan will bring failure. This is indecision. That in itself is a decision you make — but not the right one. Not the one that will work with the laws of the universe and attract what you want. Indecision and lack of planning create all-out mental wars and emotional turmoil or ambivalence. Ambivalence describes the feeling when you have both positive and negative feelings toward something or someone and are thus pulled in opposite directions: leave – don't leave; do it – don't do it; go – don't go; say it – don't say it; drink it – don't drink it; eat it – don't eat it. Eliminate these wars within yourself and you can become an effective decision maker. This takes courage; you must have the courage to believe that you can make the right decision.

The type of thoughts and ideas which, occupy your consciousness is of paramount importance in developing your Perfect Weight. Your mind is either in an orderly or a confused state. Order must prevail in your mind if you ever hope to see it manifest in your material world.

- Bob Proctor

NOTES

CHAPTER THREE

Becoming Your Vision

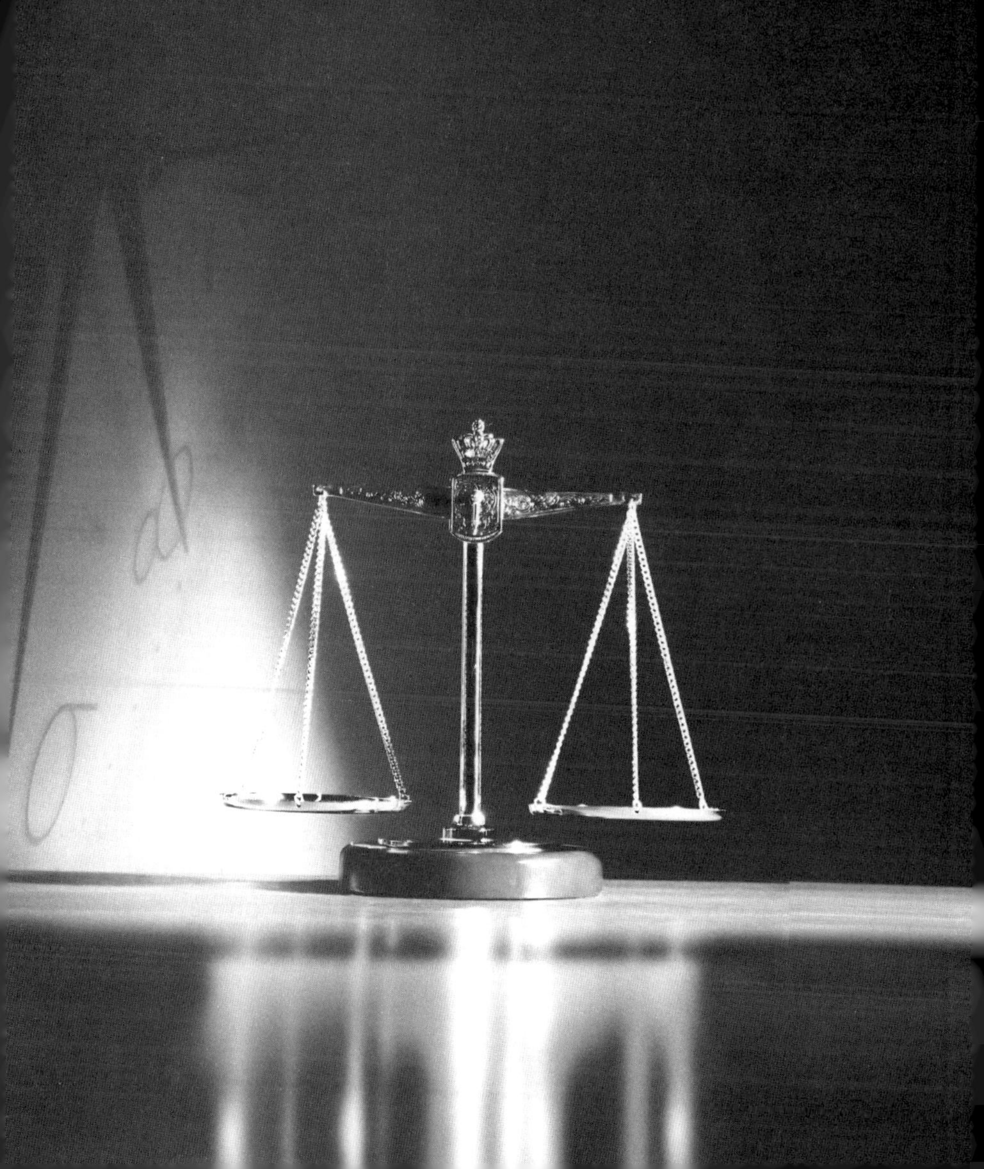

CHAPTER THREE
Becoming Your Vision

Rule your mind or it will rule you.

– Horace

If you are like many people, you've tried numerous diets and perhaps even had some success, but have slowly returned to your old habits and old weight. Why does this happen? It almost seems as if our body conspires against us at times, but the true culprit is our mindset. There is a weight that we are comfortable with. We wear it like an old sweater. It makes us feel safe and secure. We don't even know we are enabling the habits that keep it on, but we are.

People naturally resist ambiguity and uncertainty. Contemplating weight reduction is no exception. When people don't know what is to come, they get fearful and lose the ability or desire to move forward. It's ironic; we keep ourselves from succeeding, and then are confused when we don't succeed.

No matter what area of your life you want to change, you will experience this same phenomenon, whether it's weight, relationships, or career. We live our daily lives mostly on autopilot, following the deep-rooted habits we have created over time. We don't even consciously think about these habits until someone else points them out. This is often the case when people are asked how much they eat in a day. They will usually say a very normal or even small amount. However, if you monitored people's eating habits, you find that often they actually eat two to three times the amount they say they do. They aren't lying. They simply eat so much out of habit that they really don't remember everything that goes into their mouths or the amounts.

It may seem to be a very simple task to change these habits and create new ones, but it takes much more effort than you might think. By their very definition, habits are entrenched in our sub-conscious, and it takes extensive repetition to replace one habit with another. This is the time when it seems your body is fighting your efforts, but it is not your body at all, only your sub-conscious programming. How many times have you started a diet, lost 10 or maybe even 20 pounds, then watched those pounds creep right back — and maybe bring along a few friends? This is your sub-conscious mind at work. There is a range of weight that we have become accustomed to, and even if that range is morbidly obese, our minds accept this as our comfort zone. Therefore, while we may achieve success at the beginning, we lose interest or the ability to move forward. This is referred to as the **"Terror Barrier."**

When the change we want to implement starts to move us out of our comfort zone, we have feelings of uncertainty. People respond to us differently and we act differently. Fear of this unknown territory, even if it is positive, can inhibit our ability to continue because it goes against what we have come to accept as our self-image. If you believe yourself to be unattractive, then reduce your weight and start getting compliments, that's good, right? Yes and no. Of course, it is great to get positive feedback, but it also puts you in the position of gaining more attention from others; this can make some people extremely uncomfortable, as they may feel their efforts are being scrutinized. Before you know it, they regain all their weight in a sub-conscious effort to relieve the stress of being noticed.

The only way to change this behavior is to know that the change will happen and accept it as so. When you really and truly know something will happen, there is no trace of doubt, no lingering thread of skepticism. Bob Proctor uses a great analogy when referring how this knowing works. It is called the XY Factor.

THE X FACTOR is the conditioning that resonates in our sub-conscious mind. You can think of it as a habit. A good example of this might be a woman who wants to reduce her weight by 20 pounds. She's heard of the latest diets and has attempted weight reduction over the years. She thinks she knows what works for her and what doesn't. She may have learned poor eating habits from her mother and now passes her beliefs about food onto her family. This is her comfort zone.

THE Y FACTOR can be anything that represents change. It disrupts what we know and makes us uncomfortable. Now let's assume this same woman sets a target of achieving her Perfect Weight by summer. She wants to reach that target. Achieving it could change her life in great ways. It is very important to her.

It is at this point where the conscious mind makes the decision to accept Y that the X factor feels threatened. All that she has known and experienced rebels against this new idea and right away fear sets in. When fear enters the picture, logic leaves. Concentrating on that fear attracts more of the same and that goal seems even further away. This is the point where many people may give up. Doubts become overwhelming, and the sub-conscious begs to retreat back into what it has known — back into the comfort zone.

But you can fight back. Tackle your fears; only you can let them win. You know now that by concentrating on the positive goal ahead and setting those fears aside, you are imprinting new ideas into your sub-conscious. If you do this enough and concentrate on the changes you want to make and the goals you are trying to achieve, you are allowing Y to win. You are empowering your mind with new thoughts, which result in different actions. These actions produce the results that you desire.

VISUALIZATION AND THE LAW OF ATTRACTION

WE OFTEN HAVE difficulty thinking in abstract ideas. We dream in full-color movie clips! Visualization is a process that we use, even if we don't know we are doing it; it's just how we naturally think. If you think about reducing your weight, you don't think in terms of fat cells shriveling up or healthy foods being digested better by your body. You imagine how it would look and feel to be at your Perfect Weight — what new clothes you might wear or what kind of compliments you might receive.

It is important to understand how visualization and the Law of Attraction work in harmony because they function whether you know it or not, or want them to or not. The Law of Attraction states that you will attract more of whatever you focus on. This can be alarming because whatever you are thinking about repeatedly, whatever you are mulling around, grumbling about, even if only to yourself, that's visualizing — which invokes the Law of Attraction. This phenomenon starts in the thinking mind, is amplified by the emotional mind, and manifests in the body. The body, like all matter, is made up entirely of energy; thus, we all send out vibrations or energy. This energy attracts more of the same, so whatever you have been visualizing, good or bad, is reflected back to you. You have the ability to choose what you want to focus on or visualize, and therefore the vibrations you send out. Even if the goal or result you desire seems outrageous, your sub-conscious mind does not know the difference between the real circumstances and the visualized circumstances. Many people report that significant achievements can be reached after just 30 days of visualizing a goal, circumstance, or material object. This is not to say that any goal can be completely accomplished in a single month, only that you will be well on the path to achieving it, just by consciously monitoring your mental images and visualizing where you want to be.

Combining gratitude for what you already have with present-tense affirmations that allow you to visualize your goal profoundly improves your results. Focus on these images in the morning when you wake, during the day as many times as you can, and after you lay down to go to sleep at night when it's quiet and you can really concentrate. This will shift the energy you are sending out and, even more significantly, the energy you attract into your life.

I was recently talking to one of my friends and she told me that each night as she lay in bed she would say the affirmation, "I am abundant." At this time, she was having some financial problems; she had a part-time job she really enjoyed, but it just wasn't providing her with enough income to live the way she wanted to. She used this affirmation night after night, and then out of nowhere she was offered a fabulous new career with a great salary and a chance to travel and meet influential people. Bob Proctor always says you just need to know the "what," and the "how" will come. You need to know what it is that you want and then truly believe you can have it; the means for achieving it will show up when you least expect it. So decide what you want, then take steps to obtain it with affirmations, visualization, and, of course, practical steps. If your goal was to achieve your Perfect Weight, for example, use your affirmations ("I am so happy to have reached my Perfect Weight"), visualize yourself at your Perfect Weight, and eat well and exercise. Above all, truly believe that you can achieve it.

Each night she would go to bed and say the affirmation, "I am abundant."

It is not a complicated process, nor should it be difficult or seem like work. At first, you may need to put reminders on the bathroom mirror or refrigerator to focus on what you want for a moment or two each day, but after a short while, it will come naturally and you will find yourself consistently sending out positive energy — and receiving astounding results from every direction.

One of the things that trips people up when they try this is obsessing about the "how": How will it happen? What are the specific steps? How long do I wait for proof that it's happening? Let go of the how. That's the universe's job; that's why we send out the positive vibrations, so the solutions will be attracted to us.

In order to use the Law of Attraction as effectively as possible to achieve your Perfect Weight, you can follow these guidelines:

ASK FOR WHAT YOU WANT

VISUALIZATION IS MOST effective when you are very clear on what your goal or target weight will be. Since we think in pictures rather than abstract ideas, this allows you to generate a clearer picture in your mind of what you will look like once you attain your Perfect Weight. One helpful activity is to find old pictures of yourself at your Perfect Weight and put them someplace where you can see them frequently to solidify this image in your mind. If you don't have any, then look in magazines or catalogues to find pictures that show bodies that look like yours will at its Perfect Weight, and cut them out. Look at them often. You might even replace the face in the photograph with a picture of you to help you visualize yourself at your Perfect Weight.

BELIEVE IT IS YOURS

BELIEVE IN YOURSELF in the present tense, not the future. That is, think of yourself as having already received what it is you want. ***Your Perfect Weight is already yours.*** It is not a hope or a wish; thinking in the future tense leaves room for doubt. You need to adopt the unshakable knowledge that you have already achieved the goal. You must imagine, pretend, act as if, and make believe that the Perfect Weight is yours. You must see yourself moving through your daily life having achieved your Perfect Weight. Write out the number you weigh at your Perfect Weight and place it over the display of your scale, and then don't weigh yourself at all. Put your scale away out of sight where it can't contradict what you've asked for with your thoughts, words, or actions. Rather than focusing on being overweight, change your thoughts to focus on you at your Perfect Weight and allow yourself to become emotionally involved.

RECEIVE WITH GRATITUDE

IT IS ESSENTIAL to feel as good as possible about yourself while you are going through this process. You cannot attract the Perfect Weight if you constantly find flaws with your body as it is. Emotions are very powerful, and if you hold onto negative feelings about your body, you will continue to attract more of that emotion and negative thought process. You will never change your outward appearance if you constantly critique it and find flaws. In fact, you will attract more weight. Be grateful and thankful for your body, and focus on all the wonderful and great qualities you possess. As you train your mind to focus on the positive and as you feel better about yourself, you are aligning your mind with the frequency of your Perfect Weight and you are attracting it into your life.

Wallace Wattles, the author of *The Science of Getting Rich,* shares something about eating in one of his books. He recommends that when you eat you focus completely on the experience. Keep your mind in the present and experience the sensation of eating — chewing, tasting, savoring, swallowing — and do not allow your mind to drift off to other things. Try this the next time you eat a meal. When you are completely present, you will find that the flavor of the food is incredibly intense and magnificent. When you let your mind drift, the flavor virtually disappears and the body switches to autopilot. If you can eat your food in the present and focus entirely on the pleasurable experience, the food is assimilated into your body perfectly, and your mind is satiated as well as your stomach. So focus on your Perfect Weight.

MEDITATION

MEDITATION INVOLVES INTENSE concentration and contemplation, most often focusing inward but sometimes used to increase awareness of the world around us, too. Although all the major religions have used some form of meditation for thousands of years, today many people worldwide use meditation outside of any traditional religious or cultural setting for health and wellness purposes. Meditation is an extended and more intense form of visualization, and time should be set aside each day to meditate specifically on your health goals.

In meditation, you learn to focus your attention and suspend the stream of distracting thoughts that normally occupy the mind. This practice results in a state of greater physical relaxation, mental calmness, and psychological balance. Whereas the first step to changing negative thoughts or patterns is awareness, the next is practice. You must practice thinking positively, and meditating is a great way to focus your thoughts on positive emotions for an extended period of time. The Perfect Weight Program includes a morning and evening meditation practice by Dr. Patrick Porter. The complete program is available at www.bobproctorperfectweight.com.

To get the most benefit from meditation, follow these simple suggestions:

- **Choose a quiet location.** A quiet place with few distractions allows for more focus and less interruption. This can be particularly helpful for beginners. Individuals who have been practicing meditation for a longer period of time sometimes develop the ability to meditate in public places, like waiting rooms or on buses.
- **Assume a comfortable posture.** Meditation can be done while sitting, lying down, standing, walking, or any other position. Choose what is most comfortable for you and what allows you to focus without physical pain or discomfort.
- **Take calming breaths.** Stopping the ever-present train of thought in the mind is much easier said than done. A good way to begin is to take several deep cleansing breaths and think about how your body breathes. Relax your muscles from the neck down by consciously thinking about each area and relaxing it. Continue to breathe deeply. This will produce a calm, relaxed state in order to begin.
- **Allow the mind to fill with positive energy.** Allow thoughts to come and go as you remain positive and relaxed. Consider your life, as it will be when your goals

manifest in your body. Imagine even the smallest detail. Release any negative thoughts and practice gratitude for the good that you have experienced so far.

Meditation can be used on its own or in combination with other helpful movement therapies, such as yoga, Tai Chi, and Qigong — a component of traditional Chinese medicine that combines movement, meditation, and controlled breathing. The intent of using these tools together is to improve blood flow and the flow of energy at the same time.

Practicing meditation has been shown to induce some physical changes in the body, such as modulating the body's "fight or flight" response. The system responsible for this response is the autonomic nervous system, sometimes called the involuntary nervous system. It automatically regulates many organs and muscles, including functions such as the heartbeat, sweating, breathing, and digestion. The autonomic nervous system is divided into two major parts:

- The **sympathetic nervous system** helps mobilize the body for action. When a person is under stress, it produces the fight-or-flight response: the heart rate and breathing rate go up, for example, the blood vessels narrow (restricting the flow of blood) and muscles tighten.
- The **parasympathetic nervous system** regulates what some call the "rest and digest" functions. This system's responses largely complement those of the sympathetic nervous system. For example, it causes the heart rate and breathing rate to slow down and the blood flow increases to the digestive system.

Meditation works for the physical body by reducing activity in the sympathetic nervous system and increasing activity in the parasympathetic nervous system. This allows your body to respond more fully to the changes you are making in your diet and exercise routine, while also helping you focus your mind on positive thoughts.

THINKING POSITIVE IS A LEARNED SKILL

WHEN I TALK about focusing on positive thoughts and energy, I often have people tell me that they are not generally positive people and this is not natural for them. I know this comes from their ingrained, sub-conscious habits, and although you might think that "negative" people are born that way, they aren't. In truth, thinking and being positive is a learned skill.

Improving your self-image, like improving any skill, takes time and practice. Developing good self-esteem involves encouraging a positive attitude toward yourself and the world around you and appreciating your worth, while at the same time behaving responsibly toward others. Self-esteem isn't self-absorption; it's self-respect. Thinking positive thoughts about who you are and what you can become is the first step to self-respect. By working from the inside out and focusing on changing your mindset first, you can build your self-esteem; this is what will carry you through to the results. The goal of this positive thinking is to give yourself a more positive self-concept, while seeing yourself honestly and accepting yourself, and removing the internal barriers that can keep you from achieving your Perfect Weight.

She finally realized that she needed to let go of these negative beliefs and stop blaming others.

I once met with a new client — I'll call her Mary — who told me a heart-wrenching story. She told me that while growing up, she was surrounded by beautiful women: her mother was striking and her sister was your typical prom queen. They were slim, blonde-haired and blue-eyed; even the paperboy would make extra stops at their house to see their beautiful smiles. My client, on the other hand, was brown-haired and chubby as a child. Although they meant her no harm, her family always pointed out her differences. When she and her sister would argue (as all siblings do), her sister would call her fat. Her mother was obsessed with Mary's weight and had her on diets starting in her second grade. Not surprisingly, Mary grew up with a very negative self-image and ended up at a staggering 287 pounds. She carried these negative beliefs about herself for 35 years and was still using them as an excuse to remain at her current weight. Her doctor told her she needed to lose weight or diabetes was inevitable, and that her joints were already showing signs of arthritis. Mary finally realized that she needed to let go of these negative beliefs and stop blaming others. It was clear she needed to make a choice to either continue down the road of self-hatred and destruction, or make a conscious effort to forgive herself and her family and start a new way of thinking. It was only herself she had been hurting all these years.

You would be hard-pressed to find someone who hasn't suffered some type of trauma in life. Too many of us were raised in alcoholic families, bullied at school, abused emotionally, physically, sexually, or abandoned. Others have married an abusive spouse or experienced great loss or adversity. Yet at some point, we need to let go of the baggage of the past that has been dragging us down and move forward to a life of hope. We cannot change the past, but we can certainly change the future. Wouldn't now be the time to do that?

Below I have listed several positive thought strategies to help you overcome negative patterns that have prevented you from achieving your goals in the past. Choose several that you feel would help you most and incorporate them into your daily life. Write these strategies down and remind yourself to pause and change your way of thinking each time you find yourself being critical of yourself. As you become more comfortable with each new way of thinking — for example, learning not to apologize or accepting blame for another's anger — try adding a new positive thought strategy to your list.

1. **Avoid exaggerations.** Correct your internal voice when it exaggerates, especially when it exaggerates the negative. Try to avoid thinking in extreme terms such as "I always eat too much" or "I'll never lose this weight."

2. **Halt negative thoughts immediately.** Sometimes putting a stop to negative thinking is as easy as that. The next time you start giving yourself an internal critique session, tell yourself to stop it! If you saw a person yelling insults at another person, you would probably tell them to stop, wouldn't you? Why do you accept that behavior from yourself?

3. **Enhance the positive.** Instead of focusing on what you think your negative qualities are, accentuate your strengths and assets. Maybe you didn't develop enough stamina this month to run a mile, but perhaps your hard work and perseverance led to losing an additional 5 pounds. Maybe you felt nervous and self-conscious when going out to a formal social event, but you received numerous comments from friends that they were happy you joined them and had a good time.

4. **It's okay to blow it.** Maybe you did get nervous and embarrassed that you couldn't keep up in fitness class or feel bad that you gave in and ate those potato chips. It's okay. All people have weaknesses, and we all fall off the path at times or don't do things as well as we think we should. Your boss, co-workers, friends, family, mail carrier, mayor, and favorite movie star have all had embarrassing moments and setbacks. Perfection is a high goal to aim for; don't start or even end there. Make doing your best your ideal goal. Focus on what you've gained from the process and how you can use it in the future. Avoid focusing on what wasn't done or should have been done differently. Allow yourself to make mistakes and then forgive yourself.

5. **Don't bully yourself!** Don't hold yourself to standards that you wouldn't expect others to meet. It's great to want to do well, but expecting yourself to be better than the best and then punishing yourself when you fail is a vicious cycle. Using expressions like "I should have ..." is just a way of punishing yourself after the fact. Stop it. Live in the present and move forward. Don't drag the past along

for the ride. Do you remember the children's story of the little train that could? That's how you need to live your life. Keep saying to yourself, "I know I can ... I know I can ... I can ... I can!" Tell your sub-conscious you have already done it. Be kind to yourself and remember you can do this!

6. **Encourage yourself.** Instead of focusing on the negative, replace your criticism with encouragement. Give constructive suggestions instead of being critical ("Maybe if I tried to do ____ next time, it would be even better" instead of "I didn't do that right"). Compliment yourself and those around you on what you have achieved ("Well, we may not have done it all, but we did a pretty great job with what we did"). Giving praise will also encourage others to praise you, and this builds up your confidence to continue on the path.

7. **Lose the guilt.** You are not to blame every time something goes wrong or someone has a problem. Apologizing for things and accepting blame can be a positive quality — if you are in the wrong, and if you learn and move on. But you shouldn't feel responsible for all problems or assume you are to blame whenever someone is upset. Many of us know people who seem to start almost every sentence with the words "I'm sorry." I would challenge you to remove the word "sorry" completely from your vocabulary. Every time you say, "I'm sorry," you reinforce the idea that you are less than you should be in your sub-conscious mind. If you are wrong, use the words "I apologize" instead and stop telling yourself and everyone around you that you are sorry.

8. **Everyone is responsible for his or her own self.** Just as not everything is your fault, not everything is your responsibility. It's okay to be helpful, but don't feel the need to be all things (and do all things) for all people. This is putting too much of a burden on yourself — and disrespectful of those around you. Allow others to be responsible for themselves and their actions. You are not responsible for anyone else's happiness. No one can make another person happy; we are all in charge of our own emotions. Trying to force someone to feel a certain way is just wasted energy on your part.

9. **Be responsible for your feelings.** Just as you can't make other people happy, don't expect others to make you feel happy or good about yourself. And don't blame others if you feel guilty or bad about yourself. You create your own feelings and make your own decisions. People and events may set the stage for your emotions, but they can't dictate them. What others think about you and say to you can only have as much effect as you allow it to have. What's important is what you tell yourself, and how you react to others.

10. **Be kind to yourself.** People often feel perfectly comfortable treating themselves in ways they wouldn't consider treating others. Do you call yourself names like fat, ugly, and loser? Would you use those terms to describe a friend? Remind yourself that you deserve to be treated well. Do something nice for yourself sometimes, either in thought (give yourself a compliment) or action (treat yourself to a massage).

11. **Let it go.** You don't need to be all things to all people or please everyone. Give yourself permission to decide you're doing the best you can. Remind yourself when you're doing things well — don't wait to hear it from someone else.

12. **Accept compliments gracefully.** If someone says, "You look good today," don't ask yourself, "What was wrong with the way I looked yesterday?" or disagree and start finding fault with yourself. Accept compliments graciously and don't ask yourself why you haven't been complimented on something else.

13. **Let bygones be bygones.** Try not to hang on to painful memories and bad feelings as that's a surefire way to encourage negative thoughts and bad moods. Your past can take control of your present and rob your future if you let it. If you can, forgive past wrongs and move on. This includes forgiving yourself. If you have a hard time forgiving or forgetting, consider talking through your emotions with a good friend or counselor, but try not to dwell. It's important to work through things, but you can't let the past determine your future.

14. **Focus on what is possible.** Avoid "can't" thinking or other negative language. Don't be afraid to seek help in accomplishing things, but remind yourself that you don't need approval from others to recognize your accomplishments. Focus on what you're able to do. Remind yourself of all your capabilities and positive qualities.

LET GO OF THE PAST – you must look to the future to change. Stop thinking of old failures. They are the past. This is NOW. Remind yourself that this time you are focusing on the core issues that will ensure your success ***BELIEVE IT!***

On a separate piece of paper, write down the diet-related events from your past that you feel have been failures. Once you have done that, read it over once out loud. Then, in a symbolic gesture, take that piece of paper and SHRED IT, BURN IT, BURY IT, FLUSH IT.

It doesn't matter how you choose to dispose of these past failures as long as you do it. You must say good-bye, so long; you are out of my life forever! You choose what you want to say. ***In another symbolic gesture, walk to the sink and wash your hands. Now you are FREE to work toward your Perfect Weight.***

Ultimately, the only power to which man should aspire is that which he exercises over himself.

– Elie Wiesel

NOTES

CHAPTER FOUR

Fear, Anger and Food

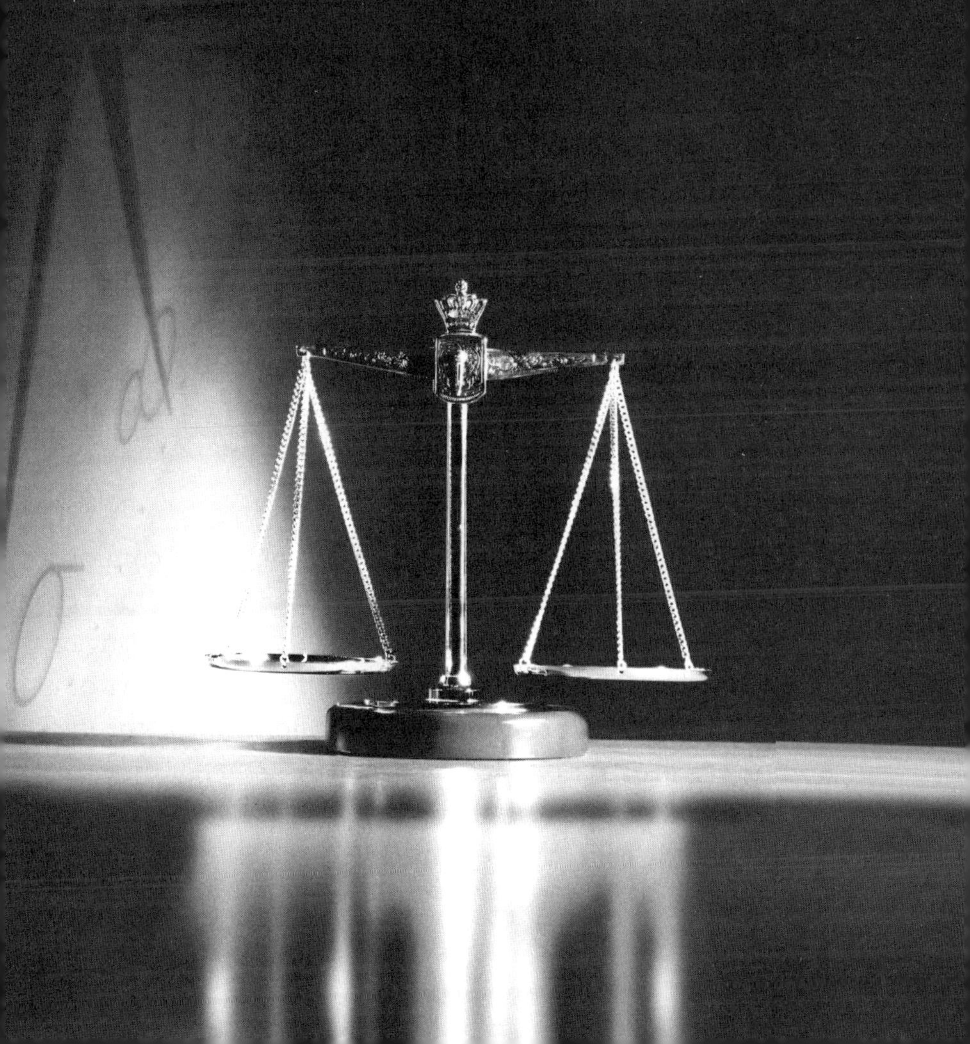

CHAPTER FOUR

Fear, Anger and Food

More die in the United States of too much food than of too little.

– John Kenneth Galbraith

Emotional eating occurs when a person consumes large quantities of food, usually high-calorie or junk foods, in response to emotions instead of hunger. Experts estimate that emotional eating causes 75% of overeating.

Many of us learn growing up that food can bring comfort, at least in the short-term. As a result, we often turn to food to heal emotional problems. Eating becomes a habit, preventing us from learning coping skills that can more effectively resolve our emotional distress. Depression, boredom, loneliness, chronic anger, anxiety, frustration, stress, problems in relationships, and poor self-esteem can lead us to overeat ... and lead to unwanted weight gain. We refer to what we eat during these times as "comfort" food. Who hasn't sat down to a bowl of chocolate fudge ice cream to make him or herself feel better? The problem is, it doesn't make us feel better, and the results from such comfort food are anything but comfortable ... especially when we go to put on our favorite jeans!

Let me tell you about Barbara. Barbara is an expert at losing weight. She should be: she's lost the same 35 pounds over and over again. She has tried all the fad diets, diet pills, and diet programs. She has been on the same weight gain/reduction roller coaster for almost 20 years. Each time she goes through the cycle of dieting, she meets her goals, then gains the weight back, each time putting on a little more weight than she lost. At 240 pounds, she fears that she will soon be over the 250 mark. Ironically, that fear contributes to her eating binges.

Barbara, like many people, is an emotional eater. Food is no longer simply fuel for her body. It has become her drug of choice, her friend, companion, comfort, and distraction from the unpleasant emotional experiences of daily life. At some point, she discovered that eating helps to medicate her pain. That association between eating and easing her emotions is reinforced daily.

There are many different triggers that can send a person into a binge of cupcakes and chips. For Barbara, loneliness is a common trigger. Having been raised in a family that says, "I love you" with food, she's come to associate eating with love. Now when Barbara feels lonely, she feeds her hungry heart. A big meal feels like a warm letter from home. It's the easiest way to fill her emptiness. Barbara told me that she has to eat bread. It is a must in her life, and something she is not willing to give up. "How else would I feel full?" she asked. The emptiness she feels is not hunger but sadness, pain, and frustration, and without knowing it she thinks and feels that bread will fill that void. It is her way of getting the support and the great big, "everything will be okay" hug she craves.

For many people, emotional eating and the resulting weight gain is a symptom of deeper issues. Dealing with any underlying emotions or problems is very important if you want to achieve your Perfect Weight. As I've already said, weight is not a function of what you put in your mouth; it's a function of why you eat. It is not until people deal with the sub-conscious causes and resolve underlying traumas that they are free to embrace new and better lifestyles. No matter how much they may rely on denial or escape, the proof of their emotional dysfunction is evident in the extra weight they wrap themselves in like armor for protection.

Take Kara. She eats when she's depressed or bored. Appetite suppressants and antidepressants can mask her problems for a while, but eventually she comes face-to-face with not liking herself and the way she lives her life. Then there's Ron. He has difficulty dealing with his marital problems. Conflict with his wife triggers a fight-or-flight (to food) response.

The situations and emotions that trigger us to eat fall into five broad categories:

SOCIAL- Eating when around other people. For example, excessive eating can result from being encouraged by others to eat, eating to fit in, arguing, feelings of inadequacy around other people, or simply associating certain people with certain foods. Thanksgiving at Grandma's is a good example. How often did Grandma give you a second helping — and because it was so delicious and because you felt you had to eat more to make her happy, you ate until you were literally sick? Or maybe your parents made you sit at the table long after everyone was finished because you hadn't eaten all of the food on your plate? You were punished for not eating.

EMOTIONAL - Eating in response to boredom, stress, fatigue, tension, depression, anger, anxiety, or loneliness as a way to "fill the void." Most people have found themselves at a party where they don't know anyone and to keep from running out the door from shyness they make the buffet table their new best friend. The sad part about this is that as you feel worse about yourself and the additional weight, you eat even more. As in the example of Barbara, this creates an endless cycle that can kill a person's self-esteem.

SITUATIONAL - Eating because the opportunity is there. For example, at a restaurant, how often do you munch on bread or chips that the servers bring to the table, whether these things really taste good or not? What about that bowl of candy on the secretary's desk you can't pass by each day? You might also associate eating with certain activities such as watching TV, going to the movies, or attending a sporting event. I often caution people about drinking alcohol, too — not only because it has empty calories, but also because drinking is

The sad part about this is that as you feel worse about yourself and the additional weight, you eat even more.

a social activity that inspires many people to habitually munch or graze, not realizing the huge numbers of additional calories they are consuming. Happy Hour with the people from the office can be devastating to the waistline!

PSYCHOLOGICAL - Eating because of negative self-worth or making excuses for eating. For example, scolding oneself for those extra pounds or a lack of willpower. Have you ever flipped past an exercise show on TV and felt a twinge of guilt ... followed by a quick trip to the fridge?

PHYSIOLOGICAL - Eating in response to your body. For example, you might have increased hunger due to skipping meals, or eat to cure a headache or other pain. How often have you gone to get a soda and a candy bar when your neck felt stiff or you needed a break from the computer?

WHY DO WE eat in response to emotions? The answer, once again, lies in the mind. We have been taught and conditioned that food is a reward; it fixes problems and heals hurts. Think back to when you were young. Did your parents ever give you ice cream or a Popsicle to help comfort you when you hurt yourself? Were you ever rewarded with a special dinner at a restaurant when you earned good grades or received a special athletic award? What about high school and college? Did you ever have a junk food marathon as a way to get through the stress of exams? Don't think for a second that this means that your weight problem is your parent's or your friends' fault. You may be conditioned, but you can change. You make your own choices.

People eat to reward themselves, celebrate occasions, and entertain others, often allowing food to become the center of social activity. They also eat to calm their nerves and comfort themselves. Many use food to numb their hearts from emotional pain; hoping food can stifle anger, rejection, or sorrow. This is especially true for people with unresolved traumas.

Lisa is a great example of this. She lives her life in fear and this fear keeps her overweight. As an adolescent, she was raped several times. The trauma of these experiences led her to believe that it wasn't safe to appear attractive. By weighing an extra 80 pounds more than her Perfect Weight, she feels more solid and secure. She also eludes male attention, which feels threatening to her. Any attempt to reduce her weight is sabotaged by this fear. Any time she gets within 30 pounds of her goal weight, her sub-conscious triggers her need for protection.

Many use food to numb their hearts from emotional pain.

Not all emotional eating has a source this intense, but the results can be the same. If you were raised to think that pretty girls aren't smart, yet knew you were very smart, it could be that you fulfilled that image in your mind and became overweight for fear of not being seen as smart or taken seriously.

Stress deserves particular attention. More than two-thirds of overweight adults report that they eat when they're stressed. When you're stressed out, you may eat extra-large portions or gravitate to junk food, reaching for a bag of potato chips when you otherwise would eat fruit.

Janice is only 10 pounds overweight, but she classifies herself as an emotional eater. Her eating is triggered predominately by stress. As a bill collector who deals with angry people all day, she soothes her frayed nerves at the end of the day with comfort foods. Similarly, Heather often grows angry at her critical, demanding, and unappreciative boss, and she deals with it by walking away — which usually means walking toward the candy machine.

BUT I'M HUNGRY!

EMOTIONAL EATERS WILL often say they eat because they are hungry and can't seem to control their hunger. Depression, sadness, anger, frustration, and hopelessness are all emotions that can be both cause and effect as the weight creeps on. These feelings are roadblocks to your success. They surface when we see people eating apple pie and ice cream drizzled with caramel sauce, or when we stand in line at the grocery store faced with the rows of chocolate bars each seemingly calling out to us, pick me, pick me! Or when our family orders a pepperoni pizza smothered with cheese. Oh, the unfairness of it all! How come we can't eat whatever we want? This misery can range from slight to intense, and may require the intervention of a physician or counselor. The feelings can be downright scary, and create a sensation of drowning, or of being trapped without a window or door for escape. Begin to manage these feelings by first not suppressing them. Acknowledge that you have them.

There are several differences between emotional hunger and physical hunger, according to the University of Texas Counseling and Mental Health Center:

1. Emotional hunger comes on suddenly; physical hunger occurs gradually.

2. When you are eating to fill a void that isn't related to an empty stomach, you crave a specific food, such as pizza or ice cream, and only that food will meet your need. When you eat because you are actually hungry, you're open to options.

3. Emotional hunger feels like it needs to be satisfied instantly with the food you crave; physical hunger can wait.

4. Even when you are full, if you're eating to satisfy an emotional need, you're more likely to keep eating. When you're eating because you're hungry, you're more likely to stop when you're full.

5. Emotional eating can leave behind feelings of guilt; eating when you are physically hungry does not.

THE PARTICULAR FOOD you reach for when eating to satisfy an emotion depends on the emotion. According to an article published in the July 2000 American Demographics by Dr. Brian Wansink, director of the Food and Brand Lab at the University of Illinois, "The type of comfort foods a person is drawn toward varies depending on their mood. People in happy moods tended to prefer ... foods such as pizza or steak (32%). Sad people reached for ice cream and cookies 39% of the time, and 36% of bored people opened up a bag of potato chips."

I'm sure you'll agree that we all eat for emotional reasons sometimes. It is when eating becomes the only or the main strategy we use to manage emotions that problems occur — and let's face it, if you're feeling a bit depressed, it's unlikely you'll reach for a carrot stick. Since emotional eating has nothing to do with actual hunger, the body probably doesn't need those calories, so they are much more likely to get stored as fat.

Not only is it important to know why you are eating, it is also important to do something about it. Following are a few tips to help you deal with emotional eating:

1. Recognize emotional eating and learn what triggers this behavior in you. You can do this by keeping a food journal that helps you keep track of what brings on your craving for certain foods.

2. Try taking a walk, calling a friend, playing cards, cleaning your house, playing golf, or doing something active or productive to take your mind off the craving.

3. When you do get the urge to eat when you're not hungry, find a comfort food that's healthy instead of junk food, such as a smoothie with fresh vegetables or fruit.

4. If you must have some comfort foods on the rare occasion, try dividing them into smaller portions. For instance, if you have a large bag of potato chips, divide it into smaller containers or baggies, and the temptation to eat more than one reasonable serving can be avoided.

5. When it comes to comfort foods that aren't healthy, like fattening desserts, think about this little tidbit of information: Your memory of a food peaks after about

four bites, so if you only have those four bites, you'll recall it as just as good an experience as if you'd eaten the whole thing. So have a few bites of cheesecake, then call it quits; you'll get equal the pleasure with fewer detrimental results.

I'M A DIET VICTIM!

I CAN'T TELL you the number of times I've spoken to someone about a weight reduction and exercise plan, only to hear excuses like these: "That's great, but it won't work for me, because my husband only wants meat and potatoes for dinner ... I'm too busy with the kids and my job, and I have no time for exercise."

A diet victim excuse is the line you tell others, and yourself, about why you haven't been successful with your health goals in the past. By and large, this is a conglomeration of misconceptions, assumptions, and denial all rolled up as one. Since I know all of us have heard or used these excuses at one time or another, let's go over a few just to get them out of the way:

"I'M JUST BIG-BONED." Hmm. Large bones make us tall, not round. The difference in skeletal structure in relation to weight is a function of height. It does not account for, nor is it an excuse for, carrying a bunch of extra pounds. You can think of it like a corn dog. If one corn dog is twice as big as the next, does that mean the stick weighs more? Probably not.

"MY FAMILY IS BIG — IT MUST BE HEREDITARY." While certain families do tend to have an easier time putting on the pounds, most often families that are overweight stay that way due to the way they have been raised to think about food, and the way they in turn pass on these perceptions to the succeeding generation. These habits are generally what cause the weight gain, not a specific gene in the family.

"MY METABOLISM IS SLOW." Although a slow metabolism does make it harder to release weight, often our metabolism slows because we have chosen not to live a healthy lifestyle. You might starve yourself all day and then eat a half-pound cheeseburger with fries. This confuses your body tremendously, and it begins holding onto food as fat. If your metabolism is slow, get up, and get moving to speed it up. This is one area you have control over, so take responsibility and stop using your metabolism as an excuse.

"HEALTHY FOOD COSTS TOO MUCH AND TASTES BAD." So, how much do your doctor's bills cost? Your blood pressure medication? How expensive will it be to have Type II diabetes due to your weight? Eating well with healthy foods does not cost nearly as much as you think it will. Just add up the money you spend on fast food, lattes, and bad habits such as tobacco and alcohol. Learning to eat healthy will actually SAVE you money and increase your life expectancy.

As far as the concept that diet food tastes bad, it merely tastes different — not bad. Your poor little taste buds have probably never had time to adjust to good food. Many people who have taken on the challenge of healthy eating and succeeded will tell you that within weeks of eating wholesome healthy food, they couldn't even stand the smell of fried chicken or French fries anymore. The body wants to be healthy and will actually develop an aversion to fast food if you let it.

"I DON'T HAVE TIME TO COOK TWO MEALS — ONE FOR ME AND ONE FOR THE FAMILY!" Of course you don't. No one does. But why would you want to cook healthy meals for you, and then continue to feed your family foods that damage their health and establish poor eating patterns that they will follow the rest of their lives? You can choose to give your family the fabulous gift of healthy eating. For the first time in history, American children are not expected to live as long as their parents because of the high rates of obesity and the amount of processed, sugar-laden foods. Consider that the next time you use this excuse.

"I HAVE TOO MUCH TO LOSE AND IT WILL TAKE TOO LONG." This is the perfectionist mindset talking. Who says there is any sort of deadline for you to meet your goal? Eating right and exercising is a lifestyle, not a one-shot marathon! Don't give yourself an artificially imposed deadline that is unrealistic. This will just make you feel worse. Commit to the lifestyle, and the goals will be met along the way.

"I AM HAPPY JUST THE WAY I AM." I have never believed anyone who was overweight that uttered this phrase. A happy person would not treat the only body he or she has so horribly. I personally am convinced that when people say this, they are really saying they fall into the next category of excuses — which is the worst one of all.

"I JUST CAN'T DO IT. I'VE TRIED AND I'M AFRAID TO FAIL AGAIN." This is the worst excuse people can use because it means they have given up. They have convinced themselves that they don't deserve to look or feel any better than they do right now. This mindset keeps more people moving toward a life of obesity and ill health than any other. The only way to ever overcome it is to focus on changing the mindset first. That is why I am spending so much time talking about the mental aspect of weight reduction before we ever hint at a food or exercise plan. If you don't have things straight in your mind, no plan will ever work. You must convince yourself that you are worth it and that you deserve to look and feel as good as you possibly can. Your very life depends on it.

BREAKING THE CYCLE

EVERY PERSON HAS a powerful capacity for healing his or her body and transforming his or her mind. To accomplish this we have to free ourselves from the past. When we release old hurts, we grow and learn to recognize happiness, and this happiness helps us stick to our goals and realize our dreams. If the past has been painful, either through diet disappointment or emotional traumas, we must stop reliving it and playing the part of the victim in the story over and over again. Every time we relive a memory, especially a past diet disappointment or an old hurt, we keep it alive in our spirits and in our bodies.

Therefore, in order to break the cycle, you have to shed the past story and create the present one. In the new story you can be determined not just to muddle through, but to thrive.

As you assume responsibility for your actions and become committed to health and fitness, you will find the solutions. Easier said than done? Well, saying it and thinking it is a good beginning. Every day you have to make a commitment to positive thinking. It is neither the win nor the loss that makes a person triumphant, only the feelings and perception you have regarding the self. Positive perception and self-affirmation is the first step to personal empowerment.

There is a Zen story of a great general who was fighting a terrible battle. His troops were outnumbered 10 to 1. The soldiers were frightened, convinced that they would lose because they were physically outnumbered. The general turned to his men and announced that he would flip his magic coin. If it fell on heads, they would fight. If it fell on tails, they would return home. The general tossed the coin in the air and it fell on heads. Believing that destiny was on their side, the soldiers fought valiantly and won. Afterwards, the second in command discussed the event with the general, delighted that fortune smiled on their little army. The general handed him the coin: it was heads on both sides. Because the men believed in their luck, they were victorious. And so it is that we make our own destiny.

In the new story you can be determined not just to muddle through, but to thrive.

In addition to positive belief and the elimination of negative self-talk, we need to live in balance. This means eating balanced meals, drinking plenty of water, and avoiding sugar, fat, and processed foods. Also, we need to get seven or eight hours sleep to reset our biological clocks daily and regenerate cells. Equally as important as what we eat is that we need to do some physical exercise every day to build up strength, stamina, and focus. When we exercise, we are empowered people of substance. We will not feel trapped or paralyzed or allow ourselves to be abused, because now we have strengthened our bones, muscles, heart, and lungs. A sound mind needs a sound body. By living in balance physically and emotionally, we shed stress. Exercise relieves stress by burning up stress hormones, releasing endorphins, and oxygenating the brain to think more clearly. Exercise also returns us to the present and away from the past!

Living in balance physically, emotionally, and spiritually is the source of energy and joy. Be kind to yourself every day and create personal time and space. If you are too busy, then eliminate some of your activities, and set realistic priorities. You have compassion for others, even your pets; make sure that you have compassion for yourself.

If you hang your swimsuit on the refrigerator door, the goodies inside will be easier to ignore.

– *The Quote Garden*

NOTES

CHAPTER FIVE

Positive is Lighter than Negative

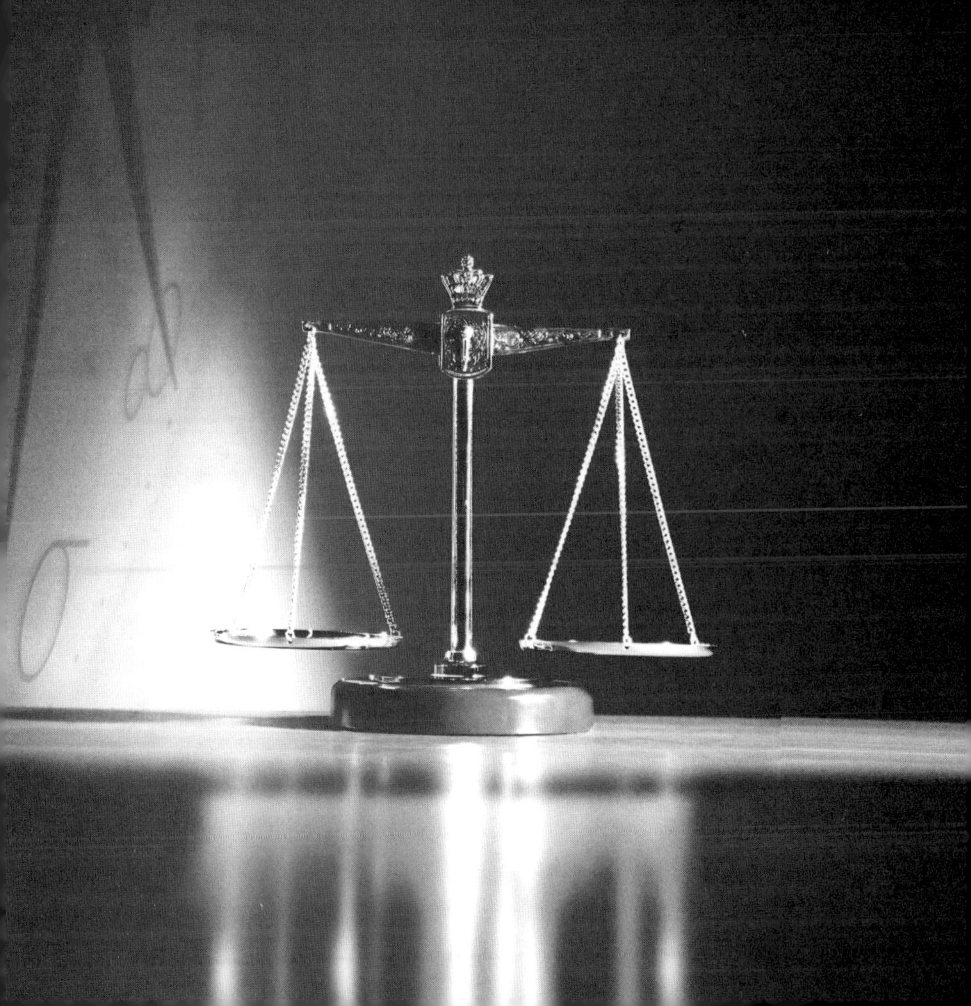

CHAPTER FIVE

Positive is Lighter than Negative

To accomplish great things, we must not only act,
but also dream; not only plan, but also believe.

– Anatole France

In the world of diet and fitness, positive thoughts are extremely important. Many people have very strong emotions and internal programming that is connected with their physical appearance. Past experiences, either positive or negative, create a stream of dialogue that runs through each person's head constantly. The tone and content of those thoughts are determining factors in reaching your weight and fitness goals.

Be aware, it is those past experiences that will cause you to doubt yourself.
Release those doubts right now; this Perfect Weight Program is different.
You don't lose weight, you release it.

-Bob Proctor

IF YOU'VE NEVER used affirmations, you might push them aside as something silly. After all it's a little self-indulgent to say things like, "I love myself" or "I believe in myself" out loud to no one, isn't it? Not at all. In a way, every thought you have and every word you say is an affirmation of some kind. All of our self-talk or inner dialogue is a constant stream of affirmations. The only reason that positive affirmations might seem awkward at first is that so many of us are so habitually negative in our thoughts and words toward ourselves that it feels strange to say something positive! We are continually affirming subconsciously with our words and thoughts, however, and this flow of affirmations colors our life experience in every moment — which makes it all the more urgent that the messages be positive.

They are dysfunctional and may be sabotaging us from achieving what we believe we want.

Our beliefs are learned through patterns that we have developed since childhood. Many of these beliefs still work well for us, but others may now be working against us. These dysfunctional beliefs may be sabotaging us from achieving what we want. For example, your parents may have rewarded you with an ice cream or some other food-related treat for passing certain milestones when you were young. Though that system of rewards worked and served you in your youth, it set up a habit of food as a reward, which can be detrimental in adulthood.

One way to overcome this embedded behavior is through the use of positive daily affirmations. Affirmations are usually short positive statements targeted at a specific sub-conscious set of beliefs, to alter and replace negative beliefs with self-nurturing beliefs. These thoughts and ideas are of your choosing, whereas many of the thoughts and beliefs from childhood were not. It is important that everything we say and think is a positive affirmation. This keeps us focused on our inner goals. It's a reminder to think consciously about our words and thoughts and to modify them to reflect our positive affirmations.

Almost every self-help program uses affirmations, even if they don't actually call them that. The reason is that they work. The more determined you are to exhibit changes in your life; the better affirmations will work for you. Repeating positive affirmations forces the sub-conscious into one of two reactions: resistance or acceptance. The bigger the issue you are trying to change in your life, the more likely it is that you will experience resistance; that is, your own sub-conscious will "argue" with you when you state your positive affirmations. Conversely, if you experience a sense of joy and well-being as you state your affirmations, your mind is instinctively responding to something it believes to be true. When you feel this emotion, you know your affirmations are working.

Repeating your affirmations with conviction and passion will weaken even the strongest resistance. Once the resistance is broken, your sub-conscious will begin to accept the new, self-nurturing beliefs. The effect can be startling, and things can change very quickly as the dysfunctional beliefs are identified and replaced by your own new inner truth.

If you find yourself experiencing serious resistance or have identified an area of trauma in your life, and your weight and health are evidence of that trauma, I strongly urge you to seek professional counseling to resolve the underlying issue first. The journey you are undertaking will assist you in letting go of the past, but having proper support around you as you go through the process will make it that much easier.

Because affirmations reprogram your sub-conscious thought patterns, they affect the way you think and feel about things. As positive thoughts replace negative ones, you will find that positive change comes easily and naturally. This will be reflected in the results you experience.

As you start out with your personal affirmations, there will be some you love and enjoy saying. These are likely to be very effective for you, and you will experience changes almost immediately. Others will make you feel uncomfortable, almost as though you are lying to yourself; this indicates resistance, and these areas may take longer to change.

If you find that a specific affirmation makes you uncomfortable, such as, "I am enjoying life at my Perfect Weight," when you know you want to release 50 pounds, you can rephrase it; saying "I am in the process of achieving my Perfect Weight." This may feel more

As positive thoughts replace negative ones, you will find that positive change comes easily and naturally.

comfortable for you. As you get more comfortable, you can switch it to the present tense.

How quickly you can resolve a resistant issue depends on the issue, how deeply held the belief is, and how determined you are to bring about change in that area of your life. Your determination to change is perhaps the most important of all. The more determined and prepared you are, the quicker those changes will come for you. Some people make significant changes in their beliefs right away, while others struggle for years. Once you are prepared to embrace and accept a change that you believe to be right for you, that change will begin to happen.

No matter what aspect of life you want to change, affirmations will make you feel better about yourself and your life. Used correctly, affirmations can change your life, affecting the way you think, reprogramming your mind, and removing the old negative beliefs that have been sabotaging you again and again throughout your life.

Various studies have demonstrated that nearly 90% of our thoughts are negative. Is it any wonder we find ourselves unable to accomplish what we want? Each negative thought or word is a negative affirmation, and these can be even more powerful than positive affirmations because we often find them easier to accept. We immediately accept the negative as true, whereas we often must be convinced of the positive. These negative thoughts feed and validate our negative internal beliefs. Under this kind of negative bombardment, most people simply do not have the strength to break free of their negative thoughts, and become hopelessly locked into their own (usually false) negative beliefs.

Thus, using affirmations is more than just chanting words or phrases. It is an entire process of becoming aware of your negative thoughts and words in everyday life, and choosing to replace them with positive ones. The more you can emotionally embrace your affirmations through your daily thoughts and words, the quicker they will work.

PERFECT WEIGHT AFFIRMATIONS

SINCE WE ARE focusing on weight and fitness, the affirmations we will talk about will concern these areas. However, this process will work for any area of your life in which you desire change. To create your own affirmations, begin by taking a piece of paper and dividing it into two sections. In one section you will put the word "weight" and in the other the word "fitness." Make a list in each section of the things that are important to you. Now take a few moments and write out several positive statements for each. The statements must be positive and in the present tense. They should focus on what you do want, not on what you don't want. For example, in the "weight" section, my affirmations might look like this:

"I enjoy eating fresh vegetables each and every day."

"The fresh vegetables I eat every day provide excellent nutrition for my body."

"By eating fresh vegetables at every meal, I am coming closer to my Perfect Weight."

Using this exercise allows you to create the affirmations that work for you, not for anyone else. Following are a few more examples to give you an idea of how they should look and feel.

AFFIRMATIONS FOR WALKING ON A REGULAR BASIS:

"I walk every day, renewing my energy and releasing stress."

"Walking every day increases my stamina and lowers my blood pressure."

"Walking every day allows my body to release stored energy moving me closer to my Perfect Weight."

THE MOST POWERFUL time for affirmations is while you are looking in the mirror. Some of the most important messages you have received have come from people who were looking at you while they delivered their messages. By looking at yourself as you state your affirmations, you increase the importance of the message to yourself. You can also see at once any flicker of your own doubt or resistance as you hear the words, see your mouth move, and note your own expression and emotion. This image impresses itself on your mind and makes your words that much more powerful. It also gives you a picture in your mind as you recall these affirmations during the day. You have an image to replay of yourself saying them over and over.

A great way of keeping your affirmations ever-present on your mind is to write them down on note cards or sticky notes and leave them in various locations, such as your bathroom mirror, refrigerator, office desk, or water bottle. Following are more examples of various affirmations to give you a start until you can create some that are more meaningful to you personally. Although most of these focus on health, there are also some general life affirmations that are important to include as well.

SAMPLE LIFE AND HEALTH AFFIRMATIONS

- I move beyond old limitations and allow myself to embrace change.
- I adapt easily to new routines that enhance my health.
- Every cell in my body vibrates with energy and good health.
- Loving myself heals my emotions.
- I nourish my mind, body, and soul.
- I choose to allow all my experiences to be joyous and loving.
- I relax into the flow of life and let it provide all that I need easily and comfortably.
- I forgive others and myself, release the past, and move forward with love in my heart.
- I love and approve of myself and am at peace with my own emotions.
- I am strong, capable, loving, lovable, and perfect, just as I am.
- I freely love and enjoy life, allowing it to flow through me.
- I allow every moment of every day to be joyous, harmonious, and loving, and I feel peace and comfort in every area of my life.

- I am enthusiastic about being active and physically fit.
- My life improves each day and is filled with more energy, vitality, and passion.
- I extend love to people on a daily basis — little by little, task by task, gesture by gesture, smile by smile, and word by word.
- I accept inspired guidance, trust the process of life, and am always safe, secure, and protected.
- I rest securely, knowing that all my needs are taken care of, that only right action is taking place in my life, and that all details take care of themselves.
- I prosper wherever I turn, and I know that I deserve prosperity of all kinds.
- I give out love and it is returned to me multiplied.
- I have wonderful relationships and am happy and at peace.
- I accept compliments from others with grace and gratitude.
- The more grateful I am, the more reasons I find to be grateful.
- I release any fear and know I will succeed.
- I know that I deserve love, and I accept it.
- I am excited to meet new people every day and embrace my new social life.

- I release any desperation and allow my body to adjust to my Perfect Weight over time.
- I attract only healthy relationships.
- I am enjoying being at my Perfect Weight.
- I choose to make positive healthy choices for myself every day.
- I choose to exercise regularly.
- I believe in myself, and others believe in me, too.
- I express my needs and feelings and reap the rewards.
- I am my own unique self: special, creative, and wonderful.
- I am at peace.
- I trust in the process of getting what I want.
- I choose love, joy, and freedom, and I open my heart and allow wonderful things to flow into my life.
- I only eat foods that nourish my healthy body.
- I easily achieve the goals I set for myself.

CONTINUED INSPIRATION

INSPIRATION IS A gift we give ourselves from within that is irresistible and uncontrolled. Unseen creative forces within each of us bring it on. How do we find it? We put ourselves in situations, frames of mind, and in the company of others that lend themselves to resounding ideas. **Make a list of people, places, and things that inspire you to reach your Perfect Weight, and write them down.** Use these to continually be inspired to stay focused on your goal.

Try to stay inspired on a daily basis. We've all rolled over in bed, seen a new blanket of snow on the ground or heard the steady pounding of rain on the roof, and had that internal argument of whether or not to exercise that day. Although you have goals in mind, your focus should be on the process. You can't allow your old programming to sneak its way back into your life. You also can't worry about what other people think, or listen to their opinions as to whether you will be successful or not. Success in achieving your Perfect Weight is not a group activity; it is different for everyone. What works for one person may not for another. Don't worry about the end results, or the how, when, and where you will achieve it. Don't worry about what others may think. Just stay on course by staying inspired — whether that comes from listening to affirmation CDs, meditating, or doing yoga. Discover what inspires you.

Those who understand The Science of Perfect Weight enjoy directing their sub-conscious minds to create new and healthy lives. With each new day they observe the small successes and continue enjoying the process. Before they know it, they're well on their way to achieving their goals. Feed your mind new positive information, and you'll start to enjoy the process as well. As you do this, you create a new habit of thinking; this will be how you create new opportunities in your life that go beyond weight and fitness.

Arguments that I often hear when I suggest this new way of positive thinking are reincarnations of the diet excuses. I worked with one client, Anne, who used every excuse in the book, including her baby — who was 14 years old by then! Many of us use the excuse that genetics and circumstances have conspired to stack the odds against us.

Never believe the odds are against you. There will be countless people telling you what you can't do. Why should you rely on their belief systems? How does anybody really know what you can and can't do? They haven't lived your life; they don't know what you may be capable of accomplishing. So how can they set the odds for or against you? They can't. Only you decide what is and is not possible, and we know that everything is possible. You must believe that. You are capable of achieving anything that you truly believe you can, so believe that you can be at your Perfect Weight, and you will be! As for Anne, once she finally let go of the excuses, she found her Perfect Weight. Standing tall at 5 feet and 8 inches, she dropped from a size 16 to a stunning size 7.

There will be countless people telling you what you can't do; they only tell you this because that's their own belief system.

"Calculating the odds" makes it seem as though life is a game of chance beyond your control. Life isn't a game of chance. Odds are irrelevant when it comes to your life and determining what you can or cannot do. So think about what you want and focus on the next step without worrying about the end result. Focus on what is going on right now. Enjoy the process.

I know many of you have had setbacks, and I realize things don't always go smoothly. It's very easy to lose faith or confidence in your ability to succeed, but all that is in the past. Begin building your healthy new life by creating a positive belief system, one that will push you to even greater success while you enjoy life every single day. And there will be plenty of days: healthy living will produce more days to enjoy in the long run by increasing your life expectancy.

Anything is possible if you have the right mindset. Once you have that in place, your conscious and sub-conscious thoughts will create the results you want day in and day out. Start working with positive affirmations and beliefs, and you'll begin implementing a new mindset that will allow you to achieve your Perfect Weight — and any other goal you set your mind to.

The good Lord gave you a body that can stand most anything. It's your mind you have to convince.

– Vincent Lombardi

NOTES

CHAPTER SIX

Creating New Habits

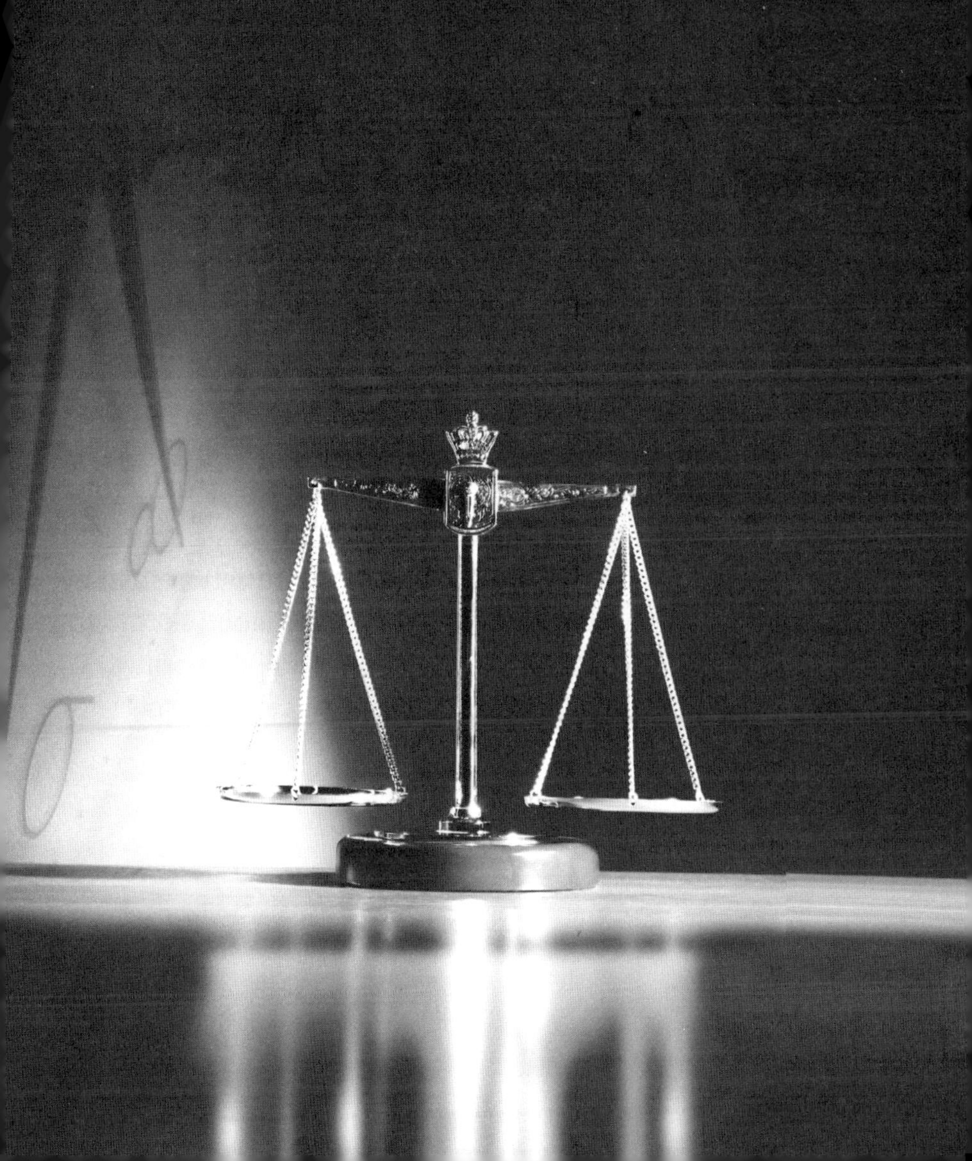

CHAPTER SIX
Creating New Habits

Great changes may not happen right away,
but with effort even the difficult may become easy.

– Bill Blackman

Achieving one's desired weight involves adopting new habits that will help you meet your goal. We often do things repeatedly, trying our best to create a new habit, only to see our efforts fall by the wayside. That's because picking up a new habit takes more than mere repetition. Provided is a step-by-step list of how to set up a new habit that will endure and serve your quest for your weight and health goals.

STEPS TO START A NEW HABIT

THE FIRST STEP is deciding which habit you wish to start. Is it perhaps a new plan to exercise everyday? Perhaps it is to walk a minimum of one mile several times a week? It is important to start yourself on the path to fitness and health with reasonable goals. You wouldn't expect to exercise for a week and then run a marathon, would you? Remember that these goals are lifestyle choices that you want to incorporate long-term, not in one-shot attempts. You must build your endurance over time. Start the habit small, and then, once it becomes a part of your daily life, increase the intensity or length.

Once you have decided on the first habit you want to start, follow these 10 steps:

1. Take a deep breath and close your eyes. Explore the motivations for this new habit. Is it to reduce your weight, get in shape, have better health, or all of the above? Picture yourself attaining the goal that this motivation brings to mind. Visualize yourself thinner, more energetic, and more able to physically do what you dream. Make this visualization as detailed as possible, and allow yourself to feel what it is like to attain it. This is getting emotionally involved with your motivation for this particular habit.

2. To enhance this visualization, write it out on a piece of paper. This helps to solidify it in your mind and also imprints it onto your sub-conscious using a different sense. Ask yourself again why this new habit would be beneficial to you, making as extensive a list as possible. Is

it something you think you "should" do? If it is a "should," you'll find that you don't care and you'll never really get this habit ingrained. However, if it is something you deeply desire from within and not something someone else thinks you should do, then it will become a part of your life. Have you ever had a friend call and ask if you'd like an exercise partner? How long does it usually last? A few days, weeks, or even months? Unless you really want this for yourself, it's very likely that eventually you will stop before it truly becomes habit since it was not inspired by your desire for good health for yourself, but something you began out of loyalty and friendship for another. You must choose the habit for yourself if it is to become part of your life.

3. Now write out what would happen in your life if you did have your new habit already in place. Would you be up to walking five miles per day? Would you be jogging instead of walking? Would you have reduced your weight substantially? How would your life be different? How would others respond to the new, more energetic, slimmer you? What would you be able to do that you are currently unable to do? What areas of your life would improve the most?

4. Choose several steps you can take each day that will assist you in creating this new habit. For the exercise example, it might be these:

- Set the alarm clock 45 minutes early.
- Have workout clothes laid out and easily accessible the night before.

- Take the dog along for companionship; the dog will benefit, too.
- Have a healthy lunch prepared the night before.
- Stock your fridge with healthy snacks you can grab quickly when you are hungry.
- Plan all of your meals in advance.
- Schedule exercise, meals, and other healthy activities into your Day-Timer or PDA.

5. Write down a date when you will start this new habit and how often you will do it. Be very specific. Choose the route you will take in the neighborhood or which gym you will go to. State exactly what you will do, as in, "I will walk three miles per day on Monday, Wednesday, and Friday each week." This is much better than simply saying, "I will exercise each week." Being specific implies a commitment to your goal.

6. Make a commitment to start. Think about what is at stake and focus again on the list you made of how it will feel, and the benefits you will receive when you incorporate this habit into your life. We have all had the experience of wanting to start an exercise program "next week"; when next week comes and goes, we just put things off, and it never happens. Make the commitment to begin — and follow through.

7. Thank yourself for participating. It is okay to be grateful to yourself, and this is a wonderful affirmation. Hearing the words "thank you" relaxes the muscles and deepens the resolve. If someone, anyone, thanks you for something, it

naturally makes you feel good. You want to keep doing it to get that praise again, so praise yourself. Soon others will see the positive changes in your life and praise you, too.

8. Notice (without judgment) when you don't follow through. Ask yourself why, but be careful not to beat yourself up over a lapse. Do you need to alter the motivation or the steps to your new habit? If so, then do it. The results you get are the product of your thinking, so if you continue to be disappointed at what you achieve, then you must be willing to ask some hard questions of yourself and change your thoughts.

9. Use your affirmations. Often people will take the affirmations they have created from the previous chapter and record them. They will then play back these affirmations each morning as they exercise. This is a great way to start the day on a positive and upbeat note while encouraging yourself to commit to your new habit.

10. Journal your progress. Journaling is a way to keep track of how far you've come and how much you've accomplished, which can sometimes be difficult for you to remember — a phenomenon we'll discuss in the next section. Journaling can be as simple as a brief paragraph noting what days you performed a certain habit or task and how it went. You can also use it to record specifics of your diet and exercise regime as well as how you are feeling as a whole and any emotional events that are occurring. It is important to do this daily. The more specific you are with your journaling, the better reference tool this will become.

HIRE A COACH

MOST PEOPLE TRYING to change a habit or achieve a new goal know that it is helpful for their success to have someone to provide support and hold them accountable. Hiring a coach who will be able to encourage you when you are having challenges and keep you focused on the goal you are trying to achieve will make all the difference for you. When you fall off track in achieving your goal, a coach can guide you back toward your plan and remind you of the goals and commitments you made. When you are focused and successful, a coach can praise you and provide you with the positive reinforcement that you need to continue to be successful. To find a coach in your area who can assist you in achieving your Perfect Weight, visit our website at www.bobproctorperfectweight.com

FOREST FOR THE TREES

HAVE YOU EVER made a big change in your life, but soon realized that those around you didn't seem to notice? Let's say you are 20 pounds closer to your Perfect Weight. You are exercising and getting fit. Do your family and friends (especially your family) start telling you how wonderful it is that you're much slimmer and more energetic?

Probably not, because they may be too close to you to see the gradual changes. This can be frustrating. For most people, making major changes to balance your life is more difficult when those changes don't seem to be noticed. It's almost like a void of reinforcement. You expect it to come, but it never does, and this creates stress.

As long as you are seeing the changes, remind yourself that eventually others will see them, too. It's just that right now they may be focusing on other things, like the fact that you are eating a completely different diet and getting up much earlier than you used to. And more than likely, they're busy focusing on their own lives, and haven't even been paying that much attention to every little thing about you. It sounds rather self-serving, but that's really how people function. We like to think we're paying attention to everything, all the time, but it often takes time to notice that something has changed. Often people who haven't seen you for a while will notice first because they have not seen the gradual changes.

How many times have you gone down a clothing size only to have someone ask if you've changed your hairstyle? If you're a parent and at one time suddenly noticed that your child is now six months old and bigger than a bread box, you understand what this means. You're so close to the situation that you can't see him/her growing. You notice it only in large increments, and even then only occasionally.

If you are going to lead the life you want and be the person you want to be, you must realize that not everyone is watching your progress as closely as you. We're not always going to find people fawning over us and telling us how much they appreciate our efforts. That kind of reinforcement is up to us. At the same time, sometimes we are too close ourselves to see many of our own changes. And we are paying attention!

The solution to this paradox is your journal. As you note the results you see and habits you form in a journal and track your progress, you can quickly see how far you've come. In this way, you can celebrate achieving milestones of health and fitness, even when they happen incrementally. Developing new habits takes concentration and concerted effort, and it can be harder when no one seems to notice or care. This is why it is so important for us to notice our own progress and congratulate ourselves. It may feel good to have someone else remark on your changes, but the best possible situation is when someone else notices something you're already giving yourself credit for.

When we are rewarded for behavior we would like to continue, that is called positive reinforcement. Positive reinforcement can work for many behaviors and in many ways. You can give yourself gold stars or write down how great you feel when you create a good health habit; both are forms of positive reinforcement and can assist you in creating the life you desire. When you want to use this technique to strengthen a behavior, it's very important that the positive reinforcement happen immediately so your mind clearly associates the reward with the desired behavior. If you were to win a marathon, but not receive your medal until weeks later, it would not be nearly as fulfilling.

Positive reinforcement can work on numerous other behaviors as well.

If there is some behavior you would like to reinforce in yourself, like exercising three times per week, you can try several methods of positive reinforcement to see what works for you. For example, immediately after returning home from your walk, give yourself praise. Throw your hands up in the air and think, "I did it!" Or give yourself a gold star on a chart you see all the time. Or give yourself points toward something special — not food, but some activity or other treat. These are very simple yet effective (and fun!) techniques to keep you on track. The important thing to remember about using positive reinforcement is that it has to be immediate and consistent, and the reward has to be meaningful in order to work.

TIPS FOR HEALTHY LIVING

FOLLOWING ARE TIPS and suggestions for improving many areas of your life through better health.

1. **Eat healthy.** The next few chapters in this book outline an eating program that will help you normalize two key areas — digestion, and your endocrine system— and help you reach your weight and fitness goals. "Eating healthy" is such a worn-out and not very specific phrase that for many of us it has lost its meaning. With all the fad diets that come and go, many people have no idea what healthy is or why certain foods are good for our bodies and others downright toxic. To live a healthy lifestyle, you must understand the chemical nature of food and how it works within your body for overall health.

2. **Maintain a healthy weight.** Obesity is at an all-time high in the United States, and the epidemic may be getting worse. Those who are overweight or obese have an increased risk for such diseases and conditions such as diabetes, high blood pressure, heart disease, and stroke. Getting your weight to a manageable level ensures a path to better overall health and energy while adding years to your life.

3. **Exercise.** More than 50% of American men and women do not get enough physical activity to provide health benefits; in other words, the most walking they do is from the refrigerator and back. For adults, 30 to 60 minutes 4 to 5 days a week of moderate physical activity is recommended. It doesn't take a lot of time or money, but it does take commitment to creating new habits. Start slowly; work up to a satisfactory level and don't overdo it. You can develop one routine, or you can do something different every day. Find fun ways to stay in shape and feel good, such as dancing, gardening, cutting the grass, swimming, walking, playing a sport, or jogging. You will find some specific recommendations later in this book such as yoga and weight training, but don't be afraid to vary your routines. Some exercise is always better than none, and once you start moving and experience the increased energy that exercise provides, it can be addictive.

4. **Be smoke-free.** Even though we all know that smoking is bad for our health, a large percentage of the population still smokes. Health concerns associated with smoking include cancer, lung disease, infertility, and pregnancy complications. Smoking triples the risk of dying from heart disease among those who are middle-aged. Second-hand smoke — smoke that you inhale when others smoke — also affects your health. If you smoke, quit today! Help-lines, counseling, medications, and other forms of support are available to help you quit, and the health benefits are immediate and substantial.

5.• **Use preventative care.** Based on your age, health history, lifestyle, and other important issues, you and your health care provider can determine how often you need to be examined and screened for certain diseases and conditions. These include high blood pressure, high cholesterol, diabetes, sexually transmitted diseases, and cancers of the skin, cervix, breast, prostate, and colon. When problems are found early, your chances for treatment and cure are better. Routine exams and screenings can help save lives, including yours. Your doctor can also monitor your overall health progress, and you can receive valuable positive feedback.

6.• **Manage stress.** Perhaps now more than ever before, job stress poses a threat to the health of workers and, in turn, to the health of organizations. Balancing obligations can be a challenge, but not taking time for yourself can cause stress overload. Protect your mental and physical health by engaging in activities that help you manage your stress, such as relaxing, eating healthy, and exercising. Visualizations and meditation can also reduce the effects of stress and allow you to react more positively.

7.• **Know yourself and your risks.** Genetics help determine some of who you are and what you might be predisposed to in the area of health. Your current habits, work, home environment, and lifestyle also affect your health and your risks. You may be at an increased risk for certain diseases or conditions because of what you do, where you work, or even how you play. Being healthy means doing some homework, knowing yourself, and deciding what's best for you.

8. **Treat yourself well.** Good health is not merely the absence of disease; it's a lifestyle. Whether it's getting enough sleep, relaxing after a stressful day, or enjoying a hobby, it's important to take time to be good to yourself. Take steps to balance work, home life, and play. Pay attention to your health, and make healthy living a part of your life.

MEAL TIME!

FOLLOWING ARE A few tips you can employ to enhance your dining experience but not your calorie intake.

1. **Pay attention.** Don't mindlessly inhale your food. Take time during meals to truly savor every bite you eat. Eat slowly. Chew each morsel and taste the food you put into your body. Turn off the television, radio, and any distractions, and allow mealtime to be a time of relaxation and enjoyment.

2. **Use a plate.** Eating directly out of the box or package can easily lead to overeating — not that we don't all do it on occasion. When you don't set aside a portion, though, that small handful of pretzels quickly becomes two, then three, and so on. Take time to put a serving of food on a plate or bowl. Eat that portion and only that portion. Many individuals find it very useful to use a small plate when they eat meals. A small plate loaded with vegetables seems like a lot of food, but in terms of calories it is a very reasonable amount. The message your brain receives is that the plate is full; therefore, it should be more than enough to eat.

3. **Use hunger as your guide.** Let your stomach tell you when you are hungry and full. Eat when you feel hungry and stop when you are satisfied. Often we let the clock guide our eating: it's noon, so it must be lunchtime. We often eat whether we are actually hungry or not. We also allow ourselves to finish an entire meal without even realizing we were full 15 minutes earlier, force-feeding ourselves out of habit. The way to stop this is through awareness and listening to our bodies. Once you have developed a lifestyle that includes a routine of healthy eating, your body will let you know when it is hungry and it will also crave healthy foods. Eating several (four to five) small meals a day is much more beneficial for your body and your metabolism than the traditional three big meals. A little saying I have reminded clients of over the years is, "Nothing tastes as good as being thin feels!"

4. **Doggy bags are the new must-have!** You don't have to clean your plate, no matter what you were told when you were 5. Save the leftovers for another meal or snack. Many people make a habit of ordering a meal or sandwich and immediately asking for half of it to be put in a doggy bag. They are more than satisfied with half a serving and also have another meal to take home. If you choose to stay at the table and talk after a meal, remove your plate so you are not tempted to keep nibbling. And absolutely no picking off someone else's plate!

5. **Slow and steady.** We all want to reduce our weight quickly, but that does not necessarily allow us to establish habits that will sustain our new weight over time. When we make overall lifestyle changes, the weight

that disappears is much less likely to return. Rapid weight reduction may feel good in the short term, but the results are rarely permanent. Usually that weight comes back, and then some. Focus on healthy living and feeling good versus losing weight! Bob Proctor reminds us that our sub-conscious will naturally want to help us "find" that which we have "lost," and this includes those pesky pounds. That is one reason why we should not focus on "weight reduction" but rather on a healthy lifestyle. This will more effectively lead you to your Perfect Weight - one that will be easy for you to maintain permanently. After all, there is no point in losing weight only to gain it back! When your focus is on a healthy lifestyle and not a number on a scale, your Perfect Weight will come!

Take care of your body. It's the only place you have to live.

— Jim Rohn

NOTES

CHAPTER SEVEN

The Perfect Weight Nutrition Plan

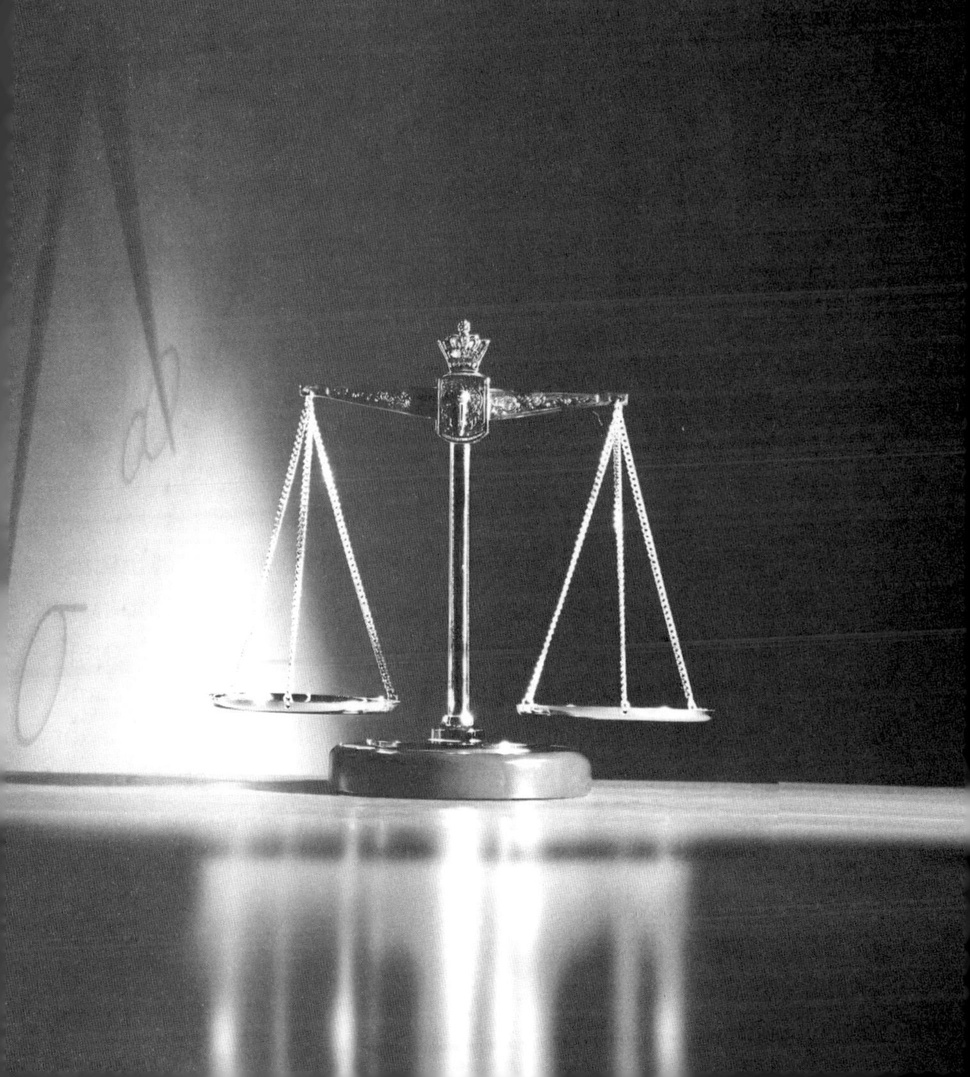

CHAPTER SEVEN

The Perfect Weight Nutrition Plan

We can reverse years of damage to our bodies by deciding to raise our standards for ourselves, then living differently. Old wounds heal, injuries repair, and the whole system improves with just a few changes in what we put into our bodies and how we move them.

– Author Unknown

The key to life long health and wellness is finding and correcting imbalances in our mind and body. We create many of our problems through negative thinking, poor decision-making, and poor dietary choices. Up until now, you have learned a lot about *your true self* and have been working on "resetting" your mind to create your Perfect Weight. Bravo! Now it is time to learn about a healthier way of eating by following The Perfect Weight Nutrition Plan.

This is not a diet. Remove the word "diet" from your vocabulary and mind. Think of this plan as a way to edit the way you eat. Diet and edit use the same letters but mean very different things. The same is true for this plan. It has many of the same strategies that you have already used to release excess fat but it is unique and will mean a new lease on life for you. This is a new way of eating that involves learning more about your body and, ultimately, about what works for YOU. You learn what to eat, when to eat it, and in what combination. Learning how particular foods influence your health is powerful information. This plan is distinctive in many ways.

No weighing and measuring foods

No pre-packaged food

No diet shakes or bars

No carb counting

No calorie counting

No constant weigh-ins

No feeling deprived

Tasty and nutritious foods

Achieve and maintain your Perfect Weight

IT IS TIME to reset your old eating habits and incorporate new healthier eating habits into your life. As Bob Proctor states, people will naturally want to find that which they have lost, and this includes weight. This is one reason why "weight loss" is not the main focus here. Our focus is on creating a healthy lifestyle. Getting back to a natural state of balance, health, and vitality will help you maintain your Perfect Weight permanently.

In previous chapters you learned how our minds function to cause us to become and stay overweight. There are physiological culprits, too, such as metabolic imbalances and inappropriate food choices. Metabolic imbalances that contribute to excessive body fat include undiagnosed hypothyroidism (low thyroid function), low stomach acid (poor digestion), hypoglycemia (low blood sugar), candidiasis (yeast-like fungus/Candida), low adrenal function (too much stress), and food sensitivities (food allergies and intolerances). Inappropriate food choices include highly processed foods, trans fats, and refined and artificial sugars.

It is important to realize that we are all bio-chemically unique. Just as we all have different outside appearances, we are different inside as well. There is no one else exactly like you. What works for you may not work for someone else. The ability to assimilate nutrients varies from person to person. People with metabolic weaknesses (e.g., poor digestion, food sensitivities) consequently have different needs for certain nutrients and must pay particular attention to food combinations or to avoiding certain foods altogether. However, there are some common threads. We all need some quantities of the same food elements (proteins, fats, minerals, vitamins, fiber, etc.). It's important, then, to discover (by reading this material) which foods will give us these essential elements.

Given the uniqueness of our bodies, it's no wonder that the "one diet fits all" approach does not work. There are many conflicting diets out there: high-protein/low-carbohydrate, low-protein/high-carbohydrate, low-fat, low-calorie ... and so on. Even among vegetarian diets there are significant differences: some recommend combining legumes with grains/nuts/seeds at the same meal to consume a complete protein, while others do not. And although every diet has probably led to a few successes, there are definitely many failures.

The Perfect Weight Nutrition Plan is specifically designed to assist in the regulation of the endocrine and digestive systems. These key factors will be instrumental in optimizing your well-being. Optimizing digestion allows us to better absorb our nutrients, and balancing our endocrine system (the system that controls hormones) will enhance and regulate metabolic activities which, in turn aids the body in functioning at peak efficiency. The Perfect Weight Nutrition Plan also works to safely reduce toxins in the body by eliminating any foods that contain refined and artificial sugars, artificial colorings, flavorings, or preservatives, refined flours, unhealthy fats, and commercialized processed dairy products.

The Perfect Weight Nutrition Plan uses a customized approach. In our Perfect Weight Program (available at www.bobproctorperfectweight.com), we start by testing for six of the top metabolic imbalances that may have prevented you from achieving your ideal weight and feeling great in the past. We do this with a questionnaire that helps uncover imbalances in your system. Being overweight, after all, is just a symptom of an imbalance in the body. We then offer step-by-step solutions that teach you what to eat, when to eat it, and in what combination.

METABOLIC IMBALANCES

1. **HYPOTHYROIDISM (low thyroid function)**
Undetected low thyroid levels are reaching epidemic proportions. The most basic thyroid test measures only the amount of thyroid-stimulating hormone being produced by the body. It takes more extensive tests to determine if the hormones are actually reaching and being properly processed by the tissues that need them. The thyroid helps regulate metabolism, and if it is not functioning well, every process in the body slows down, contributing to the many symptoms associated with an underactive thyroid. Many people with underactive thyroid also have low blood sugar surges and digestive challenges. If you have had a hard time releasing weight, are frequently constipated, and wake up in the morning tired, you should have your thyroid checked. You can do a quick check at home without a blood test. Take your temperature first thing in the morning, before you get out of bed. If your body temperature is more than two degrees lower than your normal body temperature (which may or may not be the often quoted 98.6°F), you may have an under-active thyroid. The Perfect Weight Program contains more information about this. For an accurate test, however, you do need a blood test so your physician can see your T4/T3 Ratio, TSH, and T3 uptake results. You can certainly request these tests. Usually, there is some underlying condition that causes these levels to be abnormal.

2. **LOW STOMACH ACID (poor digestion)**
We need a proper amount of hydrochloric acid in our stomach to be able to break down foods. The nutrients from these foods eventually become absorbed and the waste products eliminated. Since we suggest that you need two to three good bowel movements per day to stay at your Perfect Weight and health, if you do not have enough stomach acid to keep up with digestion, the contents of the colon may be held for days, leaving you constipated, overweight, sick, and tired. The body cannot absorb the valuable nutrients it needs while accumulating excess waste and toxins. Think about that last meal you had. How did your stomach feel afterwards? Did you feel fine, or was there an uncomfortable feeling of fullness, bloating, gas, and perhaps even pain? If so, your system may not be sufficiently processing the food you just ate. There should be none of these symptoms if you ate a meal that your system could properly digest. Poor stomach acid could be due to a number a factors, including high stress, a history of too much dairy, or even age; our ability to produce stomach acid at age 40 is half of what it was at age 18. Your flora (good bacteria) could have been reduced by recent use of antibiotics or by poor selection of foods.

3. **HYPOGLYCEMIA (low blood sugar)**
Our bodies need the sugars in our blood to be well balanced — not too high, and not too low. If blood sugar drops too low too quickly, we feel a sudden crash. We feel shaky and light-headed, and are often seized with an

intense craving for sweets, coffee, or alcohol. Responding inappropriately to this craving can put us on the vicious roller coaster ride of high and low blood sugar. Excess sugar should be stored in your muscles and liver for ready access, but metabolic imbalances can cause the sugar to be converted directly into body fat, creating more fatigue, depression, and sickness.

With respect to weight, there are two primary hormones that play a vital role in how we burn our excess fat or store it. Insulin is the key player here. When an excess of dietary carbohydrates are consumed, especially the refined kinds like white bread, white potatoes — anything refined until it's white, in fact, such as white rice, pasta made with white flour — and sugary treats, a greater amount of insulin is required to clear the bloodstream of heavy concentrations of glucose. The important point here is that insulin is our fat storage hormone. Would you believe we have our own "magic diet pill" that helps us burn excess body fat? Here's how to switch it on. Eating a meal exclusively of protein releases extra glucagon, which encourages the release of fat. This can help you shed those excess pounds. You can't survive on an all-protein diet, of course, so while an occasional one won't hurt, when looking to create your meals for the day you should, in addition to your dietary fats, add complex (instead of simple) carbohydrates along with your protein to create more long lasting energy.

THERE ARE 5 ways in which we can balance our blood sugar levels:

1) Have a high quality protein and fat source with each of your meals

2) Eat small meals every 2 to 3 hours

3) Replace all refined sugars with stevia, unpasteurized honey, real maple syrup and to learn about more, see below in the healthy sweeteners section

4) Increase your daily fiber content by eating more vegetables

5) Avoid all coffee and alcohol

4. **CANDIDIASIS (Candida/yeast-like fungus)**

Have you ever wondered why you can't control your cravings? It seems like there is a little voice in your head saying, "Eat the doughnut! Buy that chocolate bar! Get me some chips! One more cookie!" There may be. Actually, it isn't a little voice but a little fungus known in layman's terms as Candida. It thrives on sugars and starches so over time your not-so-healthy eating habits have created a nice comfortable place for it to live. Candidiasis refers to the overgrowth (more than 10% to 15%) of a yeast-like fungus. The problem occurs when there is a disturbance in their environment and Candida grows out of control, taking over the "good bacteria." If left unchecked, Candida leads to leaky gut syndrome, an undesirable condition that interferes with nutrient absorption.

Have you ever had an overgrowth of Candida and it just keeps coming back after you have treated it? It is possible that your immune system has produced antibodies against the Candida and the body has acquired a sensitivity to it. Unless this sensitivity is corrected, other measures to control Candida are unlikely to yield lasting results.

Do you continue to crave sweets and breads (sugars and starches) and even with the best intentions still give into them feeling like you are out of control? Sugars of all kinds are the natural food for the Candida organism. Since starches have to be broken down into sugars before the body can utilize them, starches also feed Candida. So do alcohol, vinegar, yeasts, and fermented foods of all kinds. Unless Candida levels are brought back to normal levels, cravings for these treats will likely continue.

5. **LOW ADRENAL FUNCTION (too much stress)**
Cortisol is a hormone that is released from our adrenal glands whenever we are under stress. This stress can be from life stresses (e.g., illness, being late for an appointment, nervousness about a job interview, screaming kids), environmental (e.g., toxins in the air, food, or water), or even self-inflicted (e.g., starving yourself in an effort to release those unwanted pounds). Knowing that high cortisol levels can lead to increased appetite and sugar cravings, it is no wonder we gain back even more weight after "dieting" or when we are under too much stress. Low adrenals are like the shocks in the car that are worn down and when you go over bumps in life we feel it. Like shocks, if the adrenals are working well we don't feel the bumps as distinctly.

How can you tell if your adrenals have been overtaxed? Perhaps you find that something that once caused you little or no anxiety, such as driving, has become a white-knuckle experience. Long-term stress can injure and even exhaust your adrenal system. Regulating the adrenal system along with eating well and managing stress can go a long way toward successful weight management.

6. FOOD SENSITIVITIES (food allergies and intolerances)

We live in a time when everyone seems always to be in a hurry. It is no wonder we are looking for quick, fast foods. In addition to "We are what we think," what we eat and absorb has bearing on our weight as well. Eating foods that are over-processed, artificially made, too high in "bad" fats, or void of any nutrition at all will eventually cause a breakdown of our bodies, leaving us overweight and sick. Take a look in your kitchen cupboard, freezer, and fridge and count the number of boxes, tin cans, and bags of processed food you stock. Where is the fresh food? What proportion of the food in your home is fresh? As we progress through this chapter we will talk more about these choices and how they affect the body.

Often a craving or addiction indicates a food allergy or sensitivity. Although people can be born with true food allergies, these can also result from inappropriate food choices — from eating foods that do not help our systems to function at peak efficiency. The most common food allergies are wheat and dairy products (particularly pasteurized cow's milk). This can be like putting low-grade fuel in a sports car; a body with these sensitivities won't run as well as if high-grade "fuel" were used. One of the many symptoms of food allergies or sensitivities is fluid retention. Discovering and eliminating the food culprits can easily result in 20 pounds of just excess water loss!

For metabolic imbalances, food allergies, and sensitivities described above, you will find your very own test in the Perfect Weight Program, available on our website, www.bobproctorperfectweight.com.

In addition to changing your mindset, there are several good ways to jumpstart these eating habits and make the overall long-term goal of good health more successful. Once we rid our bodies of toxins and excesses, our bodies will naturally start balancing themselves, and we'll know it is working because we'll feel better, have more energy, and think more clearly. How would you like to wake up each day feeling better, having more energy, and thinking more clearly? With this positive reinforcement, it then becomes easy to follow a more relaxed eating regime to keep your system in proper balance and allow your weight to release easily. Give your system a chance to help itself. Remove the highly processed foods, refined and artificial sugars and bad fats. Once your body has normalized, then you may re-introduce them in small amounts on rare occasions (e.g., celebrations, when traveling). You may also find that adding a simple-to-make green smoothie once or twice a day will make a significant impact on your health and feeling of well-being.

My friend Elizabeth could not keep her weight down no matter what she did to reduce it. She might reduce a few pounds here and there. She did reduce a good amount of weight when she was much younger but it all came back. She worked out and was physically active in her daily life; she gardened, parked her car away from the entrance of a store ... that sort of thing. She was not a couch potato. She didn't even eat potatoes. Yet she struggled with her weight. I coached her using the Perfect Weight Program and Nutrition Plan, and within two months, she was 13 pounds closer to her Perfect Weight goal. She never felt deprived. By changing her mindset, managing her blood sugars, combining her foods correctly, and choosing to fill her plate with an emphasis on eating vegetables at most meals, she found the success that had eluded her for years. Her husband and friends noticed and complimented her on the change in her body — and she felt amazing. Today she is at her Perfect Weight.

THE PERFECT WEIGHT NUTRITION PLAN

TO EXPERIENCE YOUR Perfect Weight, you must learn to use the power of your mind. You can assist this process by balancing your blood sugar and other physiological functions that relate to your weight, by eating foods that are easy to digest, and by strengthening your body to perform your day-to-day activities at your optimal best. What foods are easily digested? They are the same foods that our primitive ancestors ate before evolving into Homo sapiens (between 150,000 and 200,000 years ago) — unprocessed whole fruits, vegetables, nuts, eggs, seeds, wild game, fowl, and fish. With the advent of agriculture and animal domestication (about 10,000 years ago) our ancestors added unrefined but milled grains, legumes, and dairy to their diets — organic, of course. The grains and legumes were soaked or sprouted and the dairy was raw (e.g., cheese, yogurt, kefir). These were foods that were easy to digest, and converted blood sugar very slowly while building up the body for optimal function. There was certainly no need to diet. We aren't all hunter-gatherers anymore, but we can still forage for wholesome foods in natural food markets and farm stands today.

We consulted with a Registered Nutritionist to create the ideal way of eating for your Perfect Weight Program. Remember these four important points:

- Eat protein and a good fat along with a large portion of vegetables with each of your meals.
- Eat every three to four hours.
- Eat until you are 80% full; remember that you will eat again in three to four hours.
- Do not eat after 8:00 p.m. (the general rule is generally two to three hours before going to bed; therefore, 8:00 p.m. is ideal if you are going to bed at 10:30 p.m., which is when you should be going to bed if you wish your body to really recover and re-vitalize).

A VITAL POINT we want to reiterate is that this is a lifestyle change, not a fad diet or temporary eating plan. This is about balance. The idea is to integrate these changes into your life over time. Many people have trouble changing their habits, to help with this we've developed a simplified plan to start with. We recommend that you make the suggested changes as you assimilate the principles of each phase into your lifestyle. Creating these healthier habits may take some time, and that is fine. Just make sure you keep moving forward and picture yourself at your Perfect Weight, imagining yourself as you want to look and feel. Take each suggestion from the nutrition plan and work on applying one every day for two weeks. Once you are comfortable, add another, then another, and before you know it you will have successfully created a lifestyle with an eating and exercise regime that is easy to maintain and a natural part of your thought process. There are three phases of The Perfect Weight Nutrition Plan:

- **The Perfectly Aware Phase.** This incorporates the fewest nutritional adjustments and results in modest health rewards.
- **The Perfectly Balanced Phase.** This is the middle-of-the-road approach; it achieves additional health benefits without you having to sacrifice all the pleasures of the Perfectly Aware Phase.
- **The Perfectly Clear Phase.** This is the strictest of all phases, mimicking our ancestral eating habits to reap maximum health rewards. This would be the phase of choice for someone who wants to reach his or her Perfect Weight in the shortest length of time.

A DETAILED VERSION of the three phases of can be found in the Perfect Weight Program. Following is a list of food guidelines for the first phase, The Perfectly Aware Phase. Additional help is available in the Perfect Weight Program, available on our website at www.bobproctorperfectweight.com. In the program you will find a complete step-by-step nutrition plan in three phases to be incorporated at your own pace into your current lifestyle. It also includes a grocery shopping guide, daily food and exercise journal, a workbook, a yoga DVD, morning and evening meditations, a teaching DVD with Bob Proctor, menu plans, recipes, and more.

GUIDELINES FOR WHILE YOU'RE IN THE "PERFECTLY AWARE" PHASE

PROTEINS:

Choose one of these mainly protein foods for each meal and snack:

Protein powder (e.g. microfiltered, ion exchange, non-denatured whey isolate, hemp, or brown rice protein)

Lean cuts of meat (e.g., tenderloin, sirloin)

Lamb

Wild game (e.g., bison, ostrich, venison)

Wild and freshwater fish (e.g., salmon and trout)

Seafood

Poultry (e.g., chicken, turkey, duck)

Eggs (only organic or free range)

Dairy products, in small amounts from cow, goat, or sheep: cheese (preferably made with raw milk), e.g., raw milk, plain whole-milk yogurt, plain kefir

Nuts and seeds and their butters, preferably raw

Fermented soy products, organic, in small amounts (e.g., miso, natto, and tempeh)

Protein sources not recommended: imitation meat products (soy), processed meats containing additives and preservatives (e.g., luncheon meats, salami, bacon), commercial dairy products, including milk and ice cream, processed cheese or cheese singles, and soy milk.

Special note on soy: Unfermented soy products, including soybeans, are high in phytic acid, often called an "anti-nutrient" because it removes minerals from the body! Even in Asia, soy is used only as a condiment, not as a primary food source. Processed soy products such as tofu are rich in trypsin inhibitors, which interfere with protein digestion. Research has shown that phytoestrogens (found in soy) could be a factor in causing breast cancer, penile birth defects, and infantile leukemia. Lastly, soy is goitrogenic, which inhibits precious iodine from being absorbed by the thyroid gland, which can lead to symptoms of underactive thyroid. Fermenting or modern food processing does not remove the phytoestrogens found in soy.

CARBOHYDRATES:

Choose one of these "mainly carbohydrate" foods in moderation (exception: have as many low glycemic vegetables as you wish) to have as part of your meals and snacks throughout the day.

VEGETABLES:

For maximum results, include these with all of your meals and snacks each day.

Best choices (low glycemic): asparagus, broccoli, cauliflower, celery, cucumber, dark leafy greens (collards, kale, beet tops, spinach, Swiss chard), eggplant, garlic, green beans, leeks, lettuces, onions, peppers, radishes, summer squashes, tomatoes, and turnips.

Eat in moderation (moderately glycemic): beets, jicama, green peas, and winter squash.

Limited intake (highly glycemic): carrots, white potatoes, corn, yams, and sweet potatoes.

FRUIT:

Have once per day. Remember to always have in combination with fats and protein to help balance your blood sugar. The "ideal" fruits are those in season in your region. Limit or avoid all dried fruits.

Choose whole or fresh pressed fruits and berries. Fruits are relatively high in sugar, and even though these are naturally occurring sugars, they are still sugars. Adding less sugar to your diet makes it easier for your endocrine system to control your insulin levels, and therefore maintain or release weight. One of the goals of this program is to have you enjoy foods with little or no sweetness instead of wanting to have sweetness with every meal. You can actually wean your taste buds away from sugar until you actually crave other food flavors such as sour, bitter, or even naturally salty, like celery. Caution with those with poor digestion: When eating raw fruits, avoid combining them with meat protein. Always combine them instead with non-meat protein (e.g., protein powders, raw milk cheese, plain yogurt, nuts, and seeds). Cooked fruits may be tolerated with meat proteins.

LEGUMES:

Have in moderation due to the high carbohydrate load. Remember to combine with whole grains or nuts/seeds for your complete protein.

Why limit our legumes? Each carbohydrate food is broken down into simple sugars like glucose. The body can only use a small amount of glucose at any one time, with the remainder to be stored as body fat. Legumes include beans, lentils, peas, and peanuts.

WHOLE GRAINS:

Have in moderation, due to the higher carbohydrate content.

Your main carbohydrate source for your meals throughout the day will be vegetables. Recommended whole grains include: Amaranth, barley, quinoa, millet, buckwheat, kamut, whole oats, brown rice, rye, spelt and sprouted wheat, sprouted cereal.

DAIRY PRODUCTS:

Have in very small amounts from cow, goat, or sheep.

Recommended dairy products include cheese (preferably made from raw milk), raw milk, plain whole milk yogurt, and kefir.

NUTS AND SEEDS AND THEIR BUTTERS:

These are preferably raw.

Have in small amounts—about 12 to 15 nuts or 2 to 3 tablespoons of seeds or 1 tablespoon of nut butter.

FERMENTED SOY PRODUCTS:

Buy organically grown whenever possible.

Have in moderation. Recommended fermented soy products include miso, natto, and tempeh.

NUT AND GRAIN MILK:

Have in very small amounts or none at all. Remember to always have in combination with fats and protein to help balance your blood sugar. Nut and grain milks are a perfect substitute to pasteurized cow's milk.

Recommended nut and grain milks include brown rice, almond, coconut, and oat milk—all made without added sweeteners.

Please note: Dairy, nuts, seeds, and fermented soy products are all considered protein, carbohydrate, and fat sources. Therefore, when constructing your meals, count these particular products as all three: protein, carbohydrate, and fat.

CARBOHYDRATE SOURCES TO AVOID:

Commercial dairy products (including milk, ice cream, processed cheese, or cheese singles), soy milk, white rice, white flour and products made with it (e.g., pasta, baked goods, pastries), dried cereal (except sprouted), instant oatmeal, regular wheat (sprouted is fine), canned fruit (sweetened). As previously noted, eat these foods only in moderation: beets, green peas, jicama, winter squashes, fermented soy, legumes and whole grains. Eat these foods sparingly: carrots, corn, white potatoes, yams, and sweet potatoes, dried fruits, and dairy.

SWEETENERS:

Acceptable in small amounts: stevia (best choice), unpasteurized honey (not recommended for children or people with immune dysfunctions), agave nectar, real maple syrup, molasses, brown rice syrup, barley malt, date sugar, fruit concentrates, Xylitol, and Luo Han Guo.

Sweeteners to avoid completely: artificial sweeteners, including sucralose (Splenda®, Altern®), acesulfame K (Sunette®, Sweet & Safe®, Sweet One®), aspartame (Nutrasweet®, Equal®, Canderel®), neotame®, cyclamates, and saccharin, as well as refined sugars, including brown sugar, cane sugar, corn syrup, fructose, fructose-glucose, sucrose, maltose, maltodextrin, dextrose, and corn sugar.

HEALTHY FATS AND OILS:

For high heat/stir fry: coconut oil, fat that occurs in natural meats and poultry (fat from lot-fed or grain-fed animals is not as healthy as that of organic or free-range animals), and ghee.

For medium heat: butter, sesame oil, and grape seed oil, in addition to the ones listed above.

For low heat (not to exceed oven heat of 200-250° F) : extra virgin olive oil, in addition to the ones listed above.

For salads (do not heat): avocado oil, almond oil, pumpkin seed oil, walnut oil, unrefined flaxseed oil, hemp seed oil, hazelnut oil, and Udo's Choice™ in addition to the ones listed above.

Additional fat: avocado, olives, coconut milk, fermented soy products, nuts or seeds and their butters, and dairy (raw milk/ cheese/plain whole milk, yogurt/kefir/sour cream/raw table cream from goat, cow, or sheep).

Please note: Dairy, nuts, seeds, and fermented soy products are all considered protein, carbohydrate, and fat sources. Therefore, when constructing your meals, count these particular products as all three: protein, carbohydrate, and fat.

Fats to avoid completely: Hydrogenated or partially hydrogenated fats/oils are trans fat and are very destructive to our health. Bad fats also include corn oil, regular canola oil, vegetable shortening, partially hydrogenated oil, vegetable cooking oils, margarine, or nuts that are honey-roasted or roasted in oil.

BEVERAGES:

Water

Herbal teas (tisanes), unsweetened or with a small amount of honey or stevia

Plain and naturally flavored mineral water in glass bottles

Raw, unpasteurized vegetable juice

Raw, unpasteurized fruit juice

Certified organic coffee (limit to one cup per day), preferably decaffeinated

Black, white, or green tea (limit to one cup per day), preferably decaffeinated

Organic wine and beer (in very small amounts)

Beverages to avoid completely: Soft drinks, diet soft drinks, sport drinks, water in plastic bottles, regular fruit juice, chlorinated tap water, and ground commercial coffee.

FOOD SELECTION "CHEAT SHEET"

Foods to include in your daily diet *(These are the most nutrient-rich foods. Use organically grown versions).*	**Foods to avoid**
Green powders Probiotic cultures Sea vegetables Spinach, kale, and other dark green vegetables Broccoli Garlic Onions Wheat grass Nuts, almonds, chestnuts, coconuts (ideally previously soaked) Seeds Sprouts Sea salt Avocado Lemons and limes Whey Protein Isolate Powder Alkaline water Herbal teas Stevia	Highly processed foods (non-foods) Genetically modified foods Irradiated foods Saturated fats Sugar, Corn Syrup, Fructose, Fructose-Glucose Processed dairy "Junk" foods Peanut butter Peanuts Soybeans Dried fruit Yeast Alcohol Soda pop Sports drinks Sweets (pastry, cookies, cakes, ice cream) Artificial sweeteners White vinegar White pasta and breads

SAMPLE MENU FOR THE PERFECTLY AWARE PHASE

Note: Adjust for any metabolic imbalances.

Day 1

BREAKFAST

Berry smoothie with spinach (see recipe)

Unrefined flaxseed oil

SNACK

Rye crackers with almond butter

LUNCH

Chicken and avocado in a sprouted grain wrap

Sliced cucumber, red peppers, and celery sticks with a little hummus

SNACK

Cut-up vegetables of your choice

(e.g., radish, green pepper, snow peas, carrots, tomatoes)

Pumpkin seeds

DINNER

Wild prawns

Brown rice

Steamed broccoli, red cabbage, and cauliflower

VERY BERRY SMOOTHIE

1 cup berries or 1 whole fruit of your choice
Handful of dark leafy greens (spinach, beet tops, Swiss chard, collards, or kale)
¼ to ½ cup filtered water
2 scoops whey protein or brown rice protein or hemp protein powder

Measure amount of berries (strawberries, blueberries, etc.), or sliced apple, pear, peaches, oranges, etc. Place berries or fruit of choice in blender. Add dark leafy greens (without stems). Add filtered water. Blend until smooth (can add more or less water if you like).

Healthy Note: Only add protein powder at the very end, and mix for no more than 2 seconds to avoid overheating the amino acid profile.

Pour contents into a glass and enjoy!

For variation, try adding any of the following ingredients:
*Flaxseed powder, 1 Tbsp. (makes smoothie thicker)
*Flaxseed oil, 1 or 2 tsp.
*Cinnamon, to taste
*Nuts and seeds (raw or in a nut/seed butter form)
*Wheat germ, 1 Tbsp.
*Green foods powder, 1 or 2 scoops
A squeeze of lemon or lime juice

GETTING STARTED

To help you get started we have outlined the key points for success in The Perfect Weight Nutrition Plan.

1. Limit your consumption of sugar and white flour. Preferably you will eliminate it entirely from your diet. This means saying no to doughnuts! You must read all your food labels now. Large amounts of processed sugar cause extreme mood swings and leave you feeling listless. Opt instead for an apple or other piece of fruit (combined with a high-quality protein and fat source, as listed in the recommendations above).

2. Eliminate fried food or foods cooked in heated oils from your diet. It's amazing how often we choose fried food, even when there are healthier choices, when it is just as easy to steam veggies or stir-fry them with coconut oil rather than frying them in harmful oils. In a short period of time you will actually develop an aversion to even the smell of fried food and your stomach won't let you eat much of it either; it will literally make you feel ill.

3. Eliminate processed foods from your diet. This includes processed dinners, pizzas, junk foods, and fast food (e.g., burgers, fries, cakes, pastries, candy, chocolate, doughnuts, etc.). This is one of the hardest things to do for most people. This is not because we aren't aware that these foods are less than great on the nutritional scale, but because snacking on junk foods is deeply ingrained into our daily habits. It is also ever present in our awareness, thanks to marketing. We are surrounded by businesses offering cheap and convenient junk food, and bombarded by advertising enticing us to nibble constantly.

4. Do not eat after 8:00 p.m. This is relatively easy for most people to do. Eating late at night is usually habitual rather than necessary. When we eat very late, our bodies store a much higher percentage of the calories as fat because we are at rest. By not eating after 8:00 p.m., we ensure that fewer of the calories that are not used immediately will be stored. Remember, the general rule is to not eat two to three hours before going to bed.

5. Do not overeat. It is very easy to overeat; we do it every day. Portion sizes in America have become absolutely ridiculous. Most "meals" served by restaurants could easily feed two or more people! Begin with making it a practice to eat only half as much as you normally would, and save the remaining food for another meal. You will find that you are easily satisfied with this portion and feel better because you don't have that "stuffed" feeling that occurs when your body struggles to digest too much food at once. Eat until you are 80% full so that you are hungry in three to four hours. The time to eat again comes quickly using this strategy.

6. You will find as you focus on improving the endocrine and digestive systems along with training your conscious mind to eat as a slim and healthy person would eat, you will naturally lower your food intake and your cravings will virtually disappear. That is the reason we do not need to recommend portion sizes. There will be no weighing or measuring of food. You will eat as a thin person if you incorporate the strategies you have learned throughout this book, and the amount of food will not be an issue.

7. Limit dairy products in your diet. We have been taught from youth that dairy products are essential and necessary, and when our bodies are young and growing, this is true. Yet some people simply don't digest pasteurized cow milk products well, or they have a hidden allergy. Eliminating dairy will clear up that buildup of mucus in your throat and the pains in your gut. Women are often reluctant to do this, as they are concerned about getting enough calcium, but you do not need to worry about this if you are eating your green leafy vegetables; they are some of the best sources of calcium. If you do have concerns about calcium, there are numerous supplements that will provide any additional calcium you may require.

8. Eat fruits that are in season. Fresh fruit is a wonderful gift for your body. When it is in season, it provides the optimal nutritional value. During certain times of the year it is very difficult to get good fruit, so take advantage of it while you can. Remember that fresh fruits make an excellent breakfast food to be used in your smoothie or with nuts and seeds.

9. Always chew your food well and eat slowly. Chewing your food well aids in digestion, and also allows the body time to recognize when it is satisfied. If you eat very quickly and barely chew, then your body doesn't have as much time to send the signals to your brain telling it you are full, and it becomes very easy to overeat. Also, if food isn't chewed thoroughly, the body must produce much more stomach acid and work much harder to digest it. You also miss out on savoring the wonderful tastes that food has to offer.

10. Exercise an absolute minimum of three times per week. Exercise should include an activity that gets you sweating and breathing deeply. There are a variety of good exercises, and we always recommend that they be combined. Otherwise, you may get bored, plus you risk working only one set of muscles. Using a variety of methods including cardio, yoga, strength training, and walking allows you to stay interested and work different muscles to achieve better overall results.

11. Drink plenty of water every day. The next chapter focuses on the importance of drinking enough water to help your body perform at its best.

With this plan we feel we have given you the keys to a lifetime of healthy eating. We haven't asked you to cut anything completely out of your diet. We may strongly recommend you avoid certain foods, especially if you want to release weight or if you have a metabolic imbalance to correct. But even within these recommendations we try to suggest alternatives. For example, not all fresh fruit juice is good for everyone since some people cannot tolerate its high glycemic properties. Although we want you to be successful in achieving your Perfect Weight, we also want to teach you to make the best choices for the foods you will eat. Switching from white rice to brown, white breads to sprouted-grain breads, eggs and bacon to eggs and veggies, refined sugars to maple syrup and natural fruits ... all these should be a goal with this plan. Remember that your subconscious will seek out that which it thinks you have lost, so if we were simply to prohibit sugars, it wouldn't be long before your body would crave it in any and every form, good or bad. We'd rather give you healthy alternatives.

If the simple and easy to adopt Perfect Weight Nutrition Plan were the answer to your lifelong battle with weight, you'd change a few food selections during your day, wouldn't you? You'd think twice when faced with the choice between a salad topped with nuts and a fat-filled, sodium-laden "mystery meat" sandwich. In the cafeteria line, you'd make sure to include a good serving of green vegetables or salad along with that meatloaf surprise. You might find it easier to pour yourself a cup of herbal tea instead of that second cup of coffee, or keep a water bottle on your desk with a squeeze of lemon in it. Remember to take these kinds of small steps, and know that achieving and maintaining your Perfect Weight is a lifelong process that involves creating a healthy lifestyle to manage your weight. Your goal is to follow The Perfect Weight Nutrition Plan by creating these healthier habits so that they last a lifetime. What you put into your mouth and how you treat your body in combination with your mindset is the key that will unlock the door to your success in reaching your Perfect Weight.

My advice is to go into something and stay with it until you like it.

- Milton Garland

NOTES

CHAPTER EIGHT

The Importance of Water

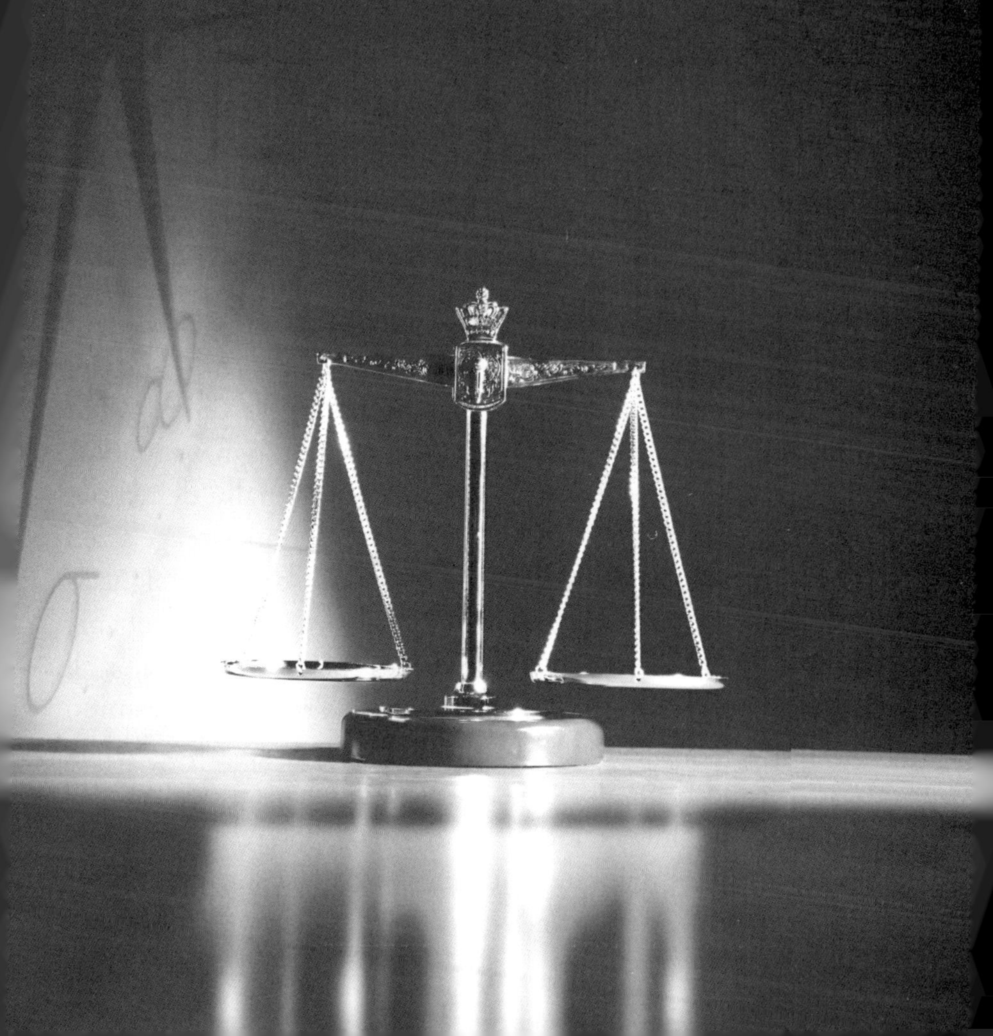

CHAPTER EIGHT

The Importance of Water

Your body is the baggage you must carry through life. The more excess the baggage, the shorter the trip.

– Arnold H. Glasgow

The human body is composed of approximately 70% water (adults 60%, babies 78%, and by the time you reach 1 year old it's 65%). Most Americans don't drink nearly enough water. Not only that, they often drink beverages that actually dehydrate the body, such as coffee and alcohol. If you are an average sized person (150 pounds/70 kilos) and don't drink at least eight 8-ounce glasses of water per day (two liters), then you probably aren't drinking enough. Water hydrates the body and helps all your bodily functions perform better. It also helps the mind function. When you are dehydrated, you experience headaches, irritation, and difficulty concentrating. Dehydration has also been shown to slow metabolism and make you retain water. In other words, not drinking enough water makes it much more difficult to achieve your Perfect Weight.

Not only is it important to drink enough water, it is also important to drink the right kind of water. We hear on the news almost on a daily basis about the impurities dissolved in our tap water. There has been much discussion, over the past few years, about the quality of the water we drink, and the effects that this may have on our health. Many health experts believe that the low quality of tap water can pose health concerns, particularly if we rely upon this as our main source of water.

These health concerns have made millions turn to bottled water with the assumption that it is better quality. Unfortunately, some bottled water is often just tap water in a pretty container. In order to get the most benefit from the water that you drink, it is important to understand that most water is slightly acidic. Pure distilled water has a neutral pH of 7.0, and most other water falls slightly below that number. It is quite easy to convert regular tap water to alkaline water by stirring in a pinch of pure sea salt. This will increase the alkalinity of your water to 8 or 8.5, which is extremely beneficial.

As the majority of the foods we eat create acid wastes in our system, it is important to drink alkaline water with a pH higher than neutral to counterbalance this process. It is also important to note that acidic water (less than pH 7) is a breeding ground of microorganisms, bacteria and viruses, that can't survive in an alkaline environment.

Acid wastes flow into the bloodstream and lymphatic system and then are transported to the liver and kidneys for detoxification processing and elimination. The pH level of our internal fluids affects every living cell in our bodies, and the effect that over-acidification can have upon the health of our bodies is immense, with a chronically acidic pH creating an extremely negative environment, which affects all cellular functions.

Alkaline water helps to neutralize acids and remove toxins from the body. It also acts as a conductor of electrochemical activity from cell to cell. Ideally, water should have a pH between 8 and 8.5, and you should be drinking no less than two liters of it daily and more optimally, three-four liters if you are exercising regularly. As you hydrate your body properly, you'll develop more of a thirst for water. We often misinterpret thirst for food cravings, so you might already have more of a thirst than you realize.

Drinking water should be one of the first things you do in your quest for good health. Since it improves the function of the body as a whole and increases your metabolism, it actually helps you reduce unwanted pounds.

It is important to take in a good portion of your daily water requirements as soon as you rise in the morning. This will allow your body and mind the best start possible for the day.

If you are someone who does not really drink much water, you may start by adding a glass of water in the morning and before or after each meal. Eventually, you will be able to progressively increase your water consumption to two-three liters per day. This will allow your body time to become accustomed to the elevated water intake. Often, during these first few weeks, you may be tempted to stop drinking because you feel like the water is running through your system within minutes. It is important to be consistent and stick to the plan. Your body needs time to balance out the new intake levels and get used to being able to function with enough water where it had to hoard water in the past. Often people who dramatically increase their water intake will lose five-seven pounds in the first week. They feel better and more energetic, experience a reduction in appetite and have noticeably clearer skin. Yes, skin eruptions can be a sign that you're a toxic waste dump inside!

One of the biggest reasons that we experience cravings for junk foods, or foods loaded with sugar and/or salt, is dehydration. Being well hydrated lessens those cravings. If you don't like drinking just plain water, add some lemon juice or a slice of lemon to it. This will also make your water more alkaline.

Few people realize that the blood collects new water supplies from the bowel.

Blood circulates and deposits water in the sweat glands, kidneys and lungs. Few people realize that the blood collects new water supplies from the bowel. Decreased hydration drops the water volume in the blood, which makes the blood thicker, reducing effective circulation.

When your circulation slows, your brain doesn't get all the nutrients or oxygen it requires as quickly as it should. The following are several things that may happen when your brain is deprived:

- You may reflexively yawn in an attempt to get more oxygen.
- You may crave sweet foods, which is your body's attempt to increase blood sugar.
- You may feel drowsy, as sleep requires less oxygen for the brain.
- You experience constipation.

By the time you experience thirst, your body is already very dehydrated. This is not the time to grab a glass of water and guzzle it to compensate. Know what your body requires and sip water regularly throughout the day. A good practice is to keep a 1-1.5 liter bottle with you during the day in your car, on your desk and on your kitchen counter. Make it a goal to drink at least two full bottles before your evening meal. This will ensure a minimum of daily hydration that is adequate.

There are numerous small health complaints that we have each day that may be eliminated or reduced simply by drinking water. Below are just a few:

- Water is essential for the body to sweat. This helps to cool the body during exercise. You can lose up to one liter of water during exercise, so it is very important to stay well-hydrated during exercise.
- Water allows for more efficient cellular repair. As cells are damaged in the course of daily life, water assists with the swift healing and repair of all cells in the body.

- Water lubricates the joints and lessens any discomfort from arthritis or back pain. It also decreases the likelihood of having arthritis.
- Water allows red blood cells to carry oxygen more efficiently, resulting in better muscular function and increased mental acuity.
- Water helps the blood cleanse toxic waste from various parts of the body and carries it to the liver and kidneys for removal.
- Water decreases stress, anxiety and depression, and allows the brain to function normally.
- Water restores normal sleep patterns and helps decrease the incidence of insomnia. (Initially you may find your sleep interrupted with regular nocturnal trips to the bathroom – that will pass – no pun intended).
- Water prevents fatigue and drowsiness.
- Water slows down the aging process and makes the skin smooth.
- Water decreases premenstrual pains and hot flashes.
- Drinking water allows you to distinguish between the sensations of thirst and hunger and to eat when you are actually hungry, which aids in weight reduction.
- Water diminishes the morning sickness of pregnancy or nausea in general.
- Water prevents the loss of memory as we age.

- Water lessens addictive urges, including those for caffeine, alcohol, and some drugs.

WHEN WE THINK of increasing the quality of our drinking water, we naturally think of water filters that are easily available at your local discount store. Make no mistake; these handy and affordable filters go a long way toward making our drinking water more beneficial and healthful. However, if you are looking for life-giving, energy-boosting nourishment from your drinking water, then these only really scratch the surface.

Transforming your water from something that simply quenches your thirst to something that you crave due to the energy and vitality it gives you is not a complex, difficult process, nor does it have to be expensive. You can greatly increase the quality of your drinking water using one of the following:

- **HOME WATER DISTILLERS.** Water distillers heat tap water electrically to boiling point. The purified condensation then drains into a clean container – leaving all of the impurities behind in the boiling chamber. Distillation kills and removes bacteria, viruses, cysts, and heavy metals. Although there is some debate about the effects of distilled water removing beneficial minerals as well as these disease-forming metals and germs, it is useful to note that the mineral content in water is so minute that one would have to drink approximately six-hundred eight-ounce glasses of water to attain the RDA of calcium and 1,800+ glasses to fulfill their daily requirement of magnesium. Distilled water also has more oxygen ions and fewer hydrogen ions, making the water far less acidic and more alkaline than other types of water.

- **WATER IONIZERS.** Water ionizers are simply products that ionize water. The water is ionized, (electrically-enhanced) by running it across positive and negative electrodes. This separates the water into alkaline (70%) and acidic (30%). This is exceptionally beneficial as the alkaline water is then used for drinking, while the acidic water can be used on the outside of the body as it is proven to kill many types of bacteria. The quality of ionized water is reputed to surpass water from any other source. For instance, ionized water is the only type of water that has a low surface tension, which allows for greater absorption of water and nutrients into the body. Some water ionizers also come with an alkalinity adjustment that allows you to set your preferred level of alkalinity. This is an incredibly useful benefit, which is unique to this type of machine. This is the system we recommend to obtain the highest quality of alkaline water. You can visit our website to learn more about water ionizers at www.bobproctorperfectweight.com.

- **OSMOSIS WATER FILTERS.** Reverse osmosis utilizes a fine membrane to filter water – known as hyper-filtration. This allows the removal of bacteria, salts, sugars, proteins, particles, dyes, and other damaging elements. Reverse osmosis uses a membrane that is semi-permeable. This allows the water to pass through while the contaminants are removed and held in the membrane. In the majority of reverse osmosis filters, this membrane is self-cleaning, allowing for the purest water to be provided. Reverse osmosis units can use between two-three gallons of water to make one gallon or they can use up to as much as 10 gallons of water or more to make one gallon of pure water. As with distilled water, reverse osmosis water is far more alkaline than tap or bottled water.

Clogged with yesterday's excess, the body drags the mind down with it.
– Horace

NOTES

CHAPTER NINE

Supplements

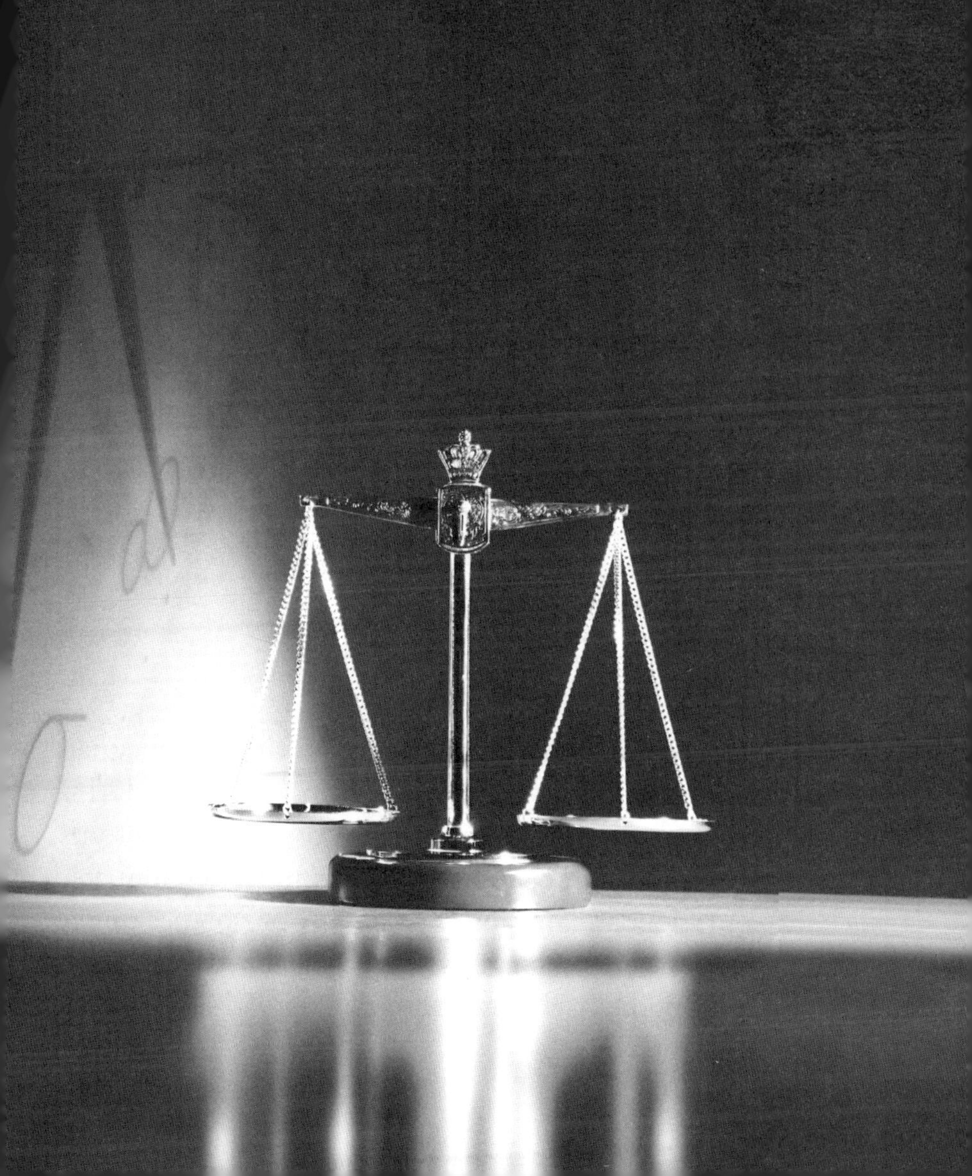

CHAPTER NINE
Supplements

The time for action is now. It's never too late to do something

– Carl Sandburg

Supplements need to be looked at as an "insurance policy" for your body. Just as you take out insurance for your car, your house, or yourself, you should take out a policy for your body.

DIGESTIVE AIDS

ONE CANNOT BE truly healthy without adequate digestion. Nutritional researchers are now convinced that autointoxication is the underlying cause of many symptoms. Autointoxication occurs when certain toxins are re-circulated back into our bloodstream slowly poisoning our bodies due to poor elimination. This explains why it is essential to our health to have 2 to 3 good bowel movements per day rather than have waste stay for days in the digestive tract, generating potentially harmful toxins. Remember, also, if you want to experience your Perfect Weight, your excess weight needs to leave your body somehow.

If you are experiencing poor digestion, nutrients are not being absorbed properly either through foods or from supplements. Your body needs to produce enough hydrochloric acid and other enzymes to properly break down proteins, fats, sugars, starches, and other carbohydrates. Low hydrochloric acid levels and enzyme deficiencies may also impair your immune function, resulting in illness.

We have half the ability to produce hydrochloric acid at age 40 as we did at age 18, which suggests that people over 40 are more likely to require some kind of digestive support. Look for a supplement that contains hydrochloric acid (to begin the breakdown of proteins) and bile (to begin the breakdown of fats). Both substances also destroy gastrointestinal parasites. Taking digestive enzymes will not suppress your own ability to produce enzymes. After eating a meal, wait a few minutes and then take your supplemental enzymes to allow your body's natural enzymes a head start, and allow the supplement to work above and beyond what your own body can handle.

PROBIOTICS (HEALTHY BACTERIA)

HAVING A WELL - functioning digestive tract is important to continued good health. It all starts with the colostrum that passes from mother to child during breast-feeding. Antibiotics, medications, cow's milk, and other difficult-to-digest substances can kill off the body's natural flora and leave an undesirable growth of Candida albicans and other unhealthful bacteria, fungus, or parasites. A diet high in simple carbohydrates, chemicals in the environment and in foods, as well as undetected allergies, also degrade the natural flora.

Healthy bacteria are natural substances that assist in keeping our immunity strong and improve digestion by stimulating peristalsis. Unhealthy bacteria do the opposite and help promote disease. Non-foods such as processed foods, hydrogenated fats, and refined sugars, are another issue. The typical American diet today consists largely of non-foods, whereas our primitive ancestors (hunter/gatherers) consumed a diet that was 80% organic and nutrient rich (consuming natural meats, vegetables, fruits, and raw nuts/seeds). Friendly bacteria help produce good lactic acid to help maintain the integrity of the large intestine. Eating poor quality foods, especially the refined and processed types, can contribute to creating a breeding ground in the colon for the unfriendly bacteria. "Friendly" bacteria in the colon produce the appropriate B vitamins, and vitamin K. They also undergo fermentation to produce lactic acid, carbon dioxide, and methane. The bacteria are also involved in the breakdown of the remaining proteins and fatty acids to their smaller components.

GREEN POWDER (GREENS)

IT GOES WITHOUT saying that it is important to eat as many vegetables as possible. One way to increase your intake is to drink vegetables in the form of a "green powder." There are many commercial powders on the market that contain highly concentrated nutrition that allow you to benefit from a multitude of vegetables, herbs, leaves, and grasses that you might otherwise find hard to include in your daily regime.

If you go to your local health food store, you will notice that green powders vary widely in the mixture of ingredients and the ratios of the blend. Check the ingredients and choose one with a variety of grasses that are nutrient dense. The vitamins and minerals in green powder are easily absorbed by the body, making this an ideal supplement. Green powder also contains fiber, amino acids, and chlorophyll, all essential for optimum health. Go green!

WHEY PROTEIN

PROTEIN IS ONE of the major building blocks of the body. Eating high-quality protein with each meal repairs and rebuilds our bodies, stabilizes our blood sugars so that we do not overeat, and helps to stimulate a fat-burning hormone called glucagon. There are three primary categories (and some subcategories or fractions) of protein powder, caseinate whey concentrate, and whey isolate. Whey protein isolate is the higher-quality protein. It's easier to digest, it's low lactose or lactose-free, and, along with a good nutritional program, may enhance cell growth and repair.

ADRENAL SUPPORT

WE ALL EXPERIENCE stress; it is how we deal with stress that is the issue here. If you find that your quality of life is compromised by your inability to handle stress, it is possible that your adrenal glands (responsible for helping you in times of stress) have become exhausted and need support. Excess stress leads to obesity, period. Excess stress also can lead to hypoglycemia symptoms, hormonal dysfunction (menopausal symptoms), underactive thyroid, and underactive digestion.

There are specific and effective supplements that may be helpful in nourishing the adrenal glands to normalize and improve their function to more optimally support you in times of stress. Nutrients that the adrenal gland requires are vitamin C, pantothenic acid (B5), potassium, rhodiola, vitamin E, and choline.

THYROID SUPPORT

THE THYROID GLAND regulates metabolism in every cell of the body. Therefore, a deficiency of thyroid hormone can affect virtually all body functions. Your thyroid produces the hormones T4 (thyroxine) and a little T3 (triiodothyronine). T4 is physiologically inactive, however, and must be converted to its active form T3 before it can begin its work in the body. Although some T3 is produced in the thyroid itself, most of the conversion occurs outside of the gland using a particular enzyme called deiodinase.

Supplements that contain nutrients to help to convert T4 to T3 may be effective in rebuilding the thyroid. Look for vitamins and minerals that work together to manufacture thyroid hormones. Nutrients that the thyroid gland needs can be found either in supplements or in foods including B-complex vitamins, vitamin E, vitamin C, iodine, and select trace minerals and amino acids. Pituitary and thyroid glandulars are also very effective and are essentially a "custom meal" used temporarily for those particular glands.

ANTI-FUNGAL AGENTS

ANTI-FUNGAL AGENTS are used to reduce the overgrowth of Candida albicans a yeast-like fungus in our bodies. Because Candida albicans is a normal inhabitant of our bodies, starving the body to eliminate it is impossible. What allows the Candida albicans to proliferate is an immune system unable to deal with it; therefore, restoring one's immunity is essential. Everyone with candidiasis can acquire a sensitivity to it. In order to bring Candida levels back to normal, one must first eliminate the sensitivity. This can be accomplished by taking a homeopathic remedy, which includes ingesting a dilution of Candida albicans every day for two months while taking additional anti-fungal agents. These include oil of oregano, garlic, grape seed extract, colloidal silver, caprylic acid, and berberine-containing plants (goldenseal, barberry, and Oregon grape).

ESSENTIAL FATTY ACIDS

ESSENTIAL FATTY ACIDS (EFAs) are called essential because our bodies cannot manufacture them and we must get them from our food. They are linoleic acid (omega-6) and linolenic acid (omega-3). Without them, we perish. EFAs are the "good fats" that we constantly hear about, and they are also a very hot research topic for scientists. More is known about them every week. Some information hasn't changed since Julius Fast wrote his book The Omega-3 Breakthrough in the late 1980s. For example, good fats compete with bad fats, so it's important to eliminate the intake of trans fats (the bad fats) while consuming enough of the good fats (listed in Chapter Seven). Also, good fats keep your high-density lipoprotein (HDL) or "good cholesterol" at its naturally higher level. One of the jobs of this HDL is to grab excess cholesterol and escort it back to the liver where it is broken down and excreted. In other words, these good fats repair some of the damage already done by the bad fats. This is very important in an age when so many people are struggling to lower their risk of heart disease and obesity. Other important factors to consider in lowering the risk of heart disease and obesity are eliminating dietary sugars, caffeine, and alcohol, and increasing foods with high fiber (i.e., vegetables low on the glycemic index; see Chapter Seven for a list) and switching from "white grains" (white bread, white rice) to 100% whole grains like whole grain spelt and brown rice. Exercising regularly is also critical to our heart health — and maintaining your Perfect Weight for life.

Essential fatty acids are necessary fats that we cannot make internally; they must be obtained through what we eat. There are two families of EFAs: omega-3 and omega-6. Omega-9 is necessary, yet called "nonessential" because the body can manufacture a modest amount on its own, provided other essential EFAs are present.

EFAs support the cardiovascular, reproductive, immune, and nervous systems. The body needs them to manufacture and repair cell membranes, enabling the cells to obtain optimum nutrition and expel harmful waste products. A primary function of EFAs is the production of prostaglandins, which regulate functions such as heart rate, blood pressure, blood clotting, fertility, and conception, and also play a role in immune function by regulating inflammation and encouraging the body to fight infection. Essential fatty acids are needed for proper growth in children as well, particularly for neural development and maturation of sensory systems, with male children having higher needs than female children.

While it is clear these EFAs are important to overall health, EFA deficiency is not uncommon in the United States. An ideal intake ratio of omega-6 to omega-3 fatty acids is between 1:1 and 4:1, with most Americans only obtaining a ratio between 10:1 and 25:1. One tablespoon of flaxseed oil can provide an adequate amount, or larger amounts of other omega-rich foods. Because high heat destroys these acids, cooking in omega-rich oils or eating cooked omega-rich fish is unlikely to provide a sufficient amount. A link has been suggested between EFA deficiency and omega-6/omega-3 imbalance and such health conditions as heart attacks, cancer, insulin resistance, asthma, lupus, schizophrenia, depression, postpartum depression, accelerated aging, stroke, obesity, diabetes, arthritis, ADHD, and Alzheimer's disease.

OMEGA-3 (LINOLENIC ACID)

OMEGA-3S ARE used in the formation of cell walls, making them supple and flexible and improving circulation and oxygen uptake with proper red blood cell flexibility and function. Omega-3 deficiencies have been linked to decreased memory and mental abilities, tingling sensation of the nerves, poor vision, increased tendency to form blood clots, diminished immune function, increased triglycerides and "bad" cholesterol (LDL) concentrations, impaired membrane function, hypertension, irregular heart beat, learning disorders, menopausal discomfort, itchiness on the front of the lower leg(s), and growth problems. Omega-3 is found in the following foods: flaxseed oil (flaxseed oil has the highest omega-3 content of any food), flaxseeds, flaxseed meal, hempseed oil, hempseeds, walnuts, pumpkin seeds, Brazil nuts, butternuts, pecans, hazelnuts, sesame seeds, avocados, some dark leafy green vegetables (kale, spinach, purslane, mustard greens, collards, etc.), kiwis, wheat germ oil, salmon, mackerel, lake trout, sardines, anchovies, albacore tuna, and others.

One tablespoon per day of flaxseed oil should provide the recommended daily adult portion of omega-3, although time-released effects of consuming nuts and other omega-rich foods is being studied, and may be more beneficial than a once-daily oil intake. Flaxseed oil used for dietary supplementation should be kept in the refrigerator or freezer, and purchased from a supplier who refrigerates the liquid as well.

Canola oil is often used as a less-expensive alternative to the healthier virgin olive and grape seed oils. Although canola has at least some omega-3 content, some supermarket varieties of canola oil have been refined and processed with chemicals and heat, which destroys much of its omega-3. Cold-pressed, unrefined canola oil is a healthier type of canola (sometimes pricier than virgin olive oil), and found primarily in health food stores and specialty markets. The word "canola" is derived from "Canadian oil, low acid" as canola was developed in Canada from the rapeseed plant. Rape is a plant in the mustard family, and its rapeseed oil has at times been illegally blended with olive oil, particularly in Europe, to cheapen olive oil production costs. Although pure rapeseed oil is high in omega-3, it can make humans seriously ill if enough is consumed, and olive oil cheapened with rapeseed oil has a history of severely sickening its consumers.

Canola was developed to eliminate chemicals toxic to humans in rapeseed oil (glucosinolates and erucic acid), thus creating an inexpensive oil with omega-3. Unlike olive and flaxseed oil, both known to the ancients and used for centuries, canola is a more recent introduction, and its long-term effects on humans are not yet known.

Unripe flaxseeds contain hydrogen cyanide, toxic in large quantities, and home gardeners should be cautious if trying to grow flax. The seeds must be ripe before harvesting. If attempting to grow flax at home, consult an experienced grower.

OMEGA-6 (LINOLEIC ACID)

LINOLEIC ACID IS the primary omega-6 fatty acid. Some omega-6s improve diabetes, rheumatoid arthritis, PMS, skin disorders (e.g., psoriasis and eczema), and aid in cancer treatment. Although most people obtain an excess of omega-6, it may not be converted into a usable form due to metabolic problems caused by diets rich in sugar, alcohol, or trans fats, as well as smoking, pollution, stress, aging, viral infections, and other illnesses like diabetes. It is best to eliminate these factors when possible, but some prefer to supplement with foods rich in omega-6 such as borage oil, black currant seed oil, nuts, eggs, whole grains, or evening primrose oil.

Omega-6 is found in the following foods: flaxseed oil, flaxseeds, flaxseed meal, hempseed oil, hempseeds, grape seed oil, pumpkin seeds, pine nuts, pistachio nuts, sunflower seeds (raw), olive oil, olives, borage oil, evening primrose oil, black currant seed oil, chestnut oil and chicken, among many others. Avoid refined and hydrogenated versions of these foods. Corn, safflower, sunflower, soybean, and cottonseed oils are also sources of omega-6, but are refined and may be nutrient-deficient as sold in stores.

If you want what you do not have, you must do what you have not done.

– Unknown Author

NOTES

CHAPTER TEN

Get Moving!

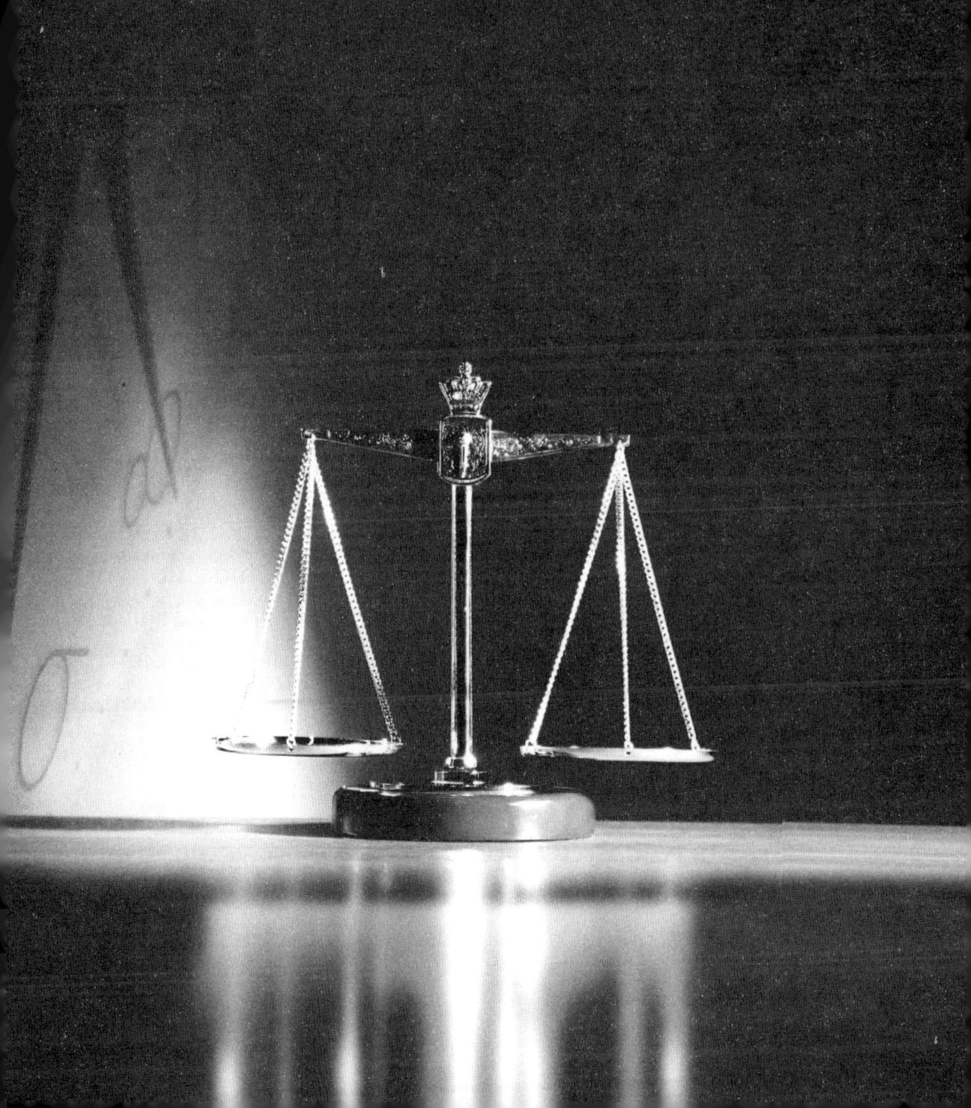

CHAPTER TEN
Get Moving!

The starting point of all achievement is desire. Keep this constantly in mind. Strengthen your desire! Weak desire brings weak results, just as a small amount of fire makes a small amount of heat.

– Author Unknown

Many people blame their inability to achieve their Perfect Weight on a weak metabolism. It's important to understand not only what metabolism is, but also what it isn't. Metabolism is the chemical process whereby your body converts food and other things into energy (calories). Whether you are eating, drinking, sleeping, cleaning, or exercising, your body is constantly burning calories to keep you going.

Metabolism is affected by your particular body composition. By body composition, I mean the amount of muscle you have versus the amount of fat. Muscle uses more calories to maintain itself than fat. People who are more muscular (and have a lower percentage of body fat) are said to have a higher metabolism than others who are less muscular. For example, let's say you have two people who are the exact same height and weight. One exercises on a regular basis with weights in addition to doing aerobic exercise, and has a low percentage of body fat. The other never exercises and has a higher percentage of body fat. The person who exercises will have a higher metabolism than the person who doesn't. What this means is that the first person's body will burn more calories to sustain itself than the second one.

People often ask how they can increase their metabolism, and it's really quite simple — so simple, in fact, that many people don't believe it. All they have to do is exercise and stop dieting. It is important not to stop eating, as the body needs fuel to burn. Do not skip any meals, do enjoy healthy snacks between meals, and drink plenty of water.

You can increase your muscle mass by doing some type of resistance workout such as lifting weights. You can also decrease your level of body fat by doing some type of cardio exercise at least three days a week for longer than 20 minutes. Refer to the "SSS Training System" philosophy in the Perfect Weight Program for details. By cardio exercise, I mean an activity that will increase your heart rate and keep it there for the duration of the exercise session (e.g., walking, jogging, step aerobics, hi/low aerobics, biking, swimming).

Often individuals who never had a weight problem when they were young begin gaining as they age. After age 30, your body tends to lose its muscle tone. If your activity level stays the same and the number of calories you eat stays the same, you will gain weight; your metabolism will have slowed down due to this loss of muscle tone, and your body will therefore burn fewer of the calories you are taking in. You can forestall this natural tendency through exercise. If you work out with weights and do some type of cardio activity on a regular basis, you probably won't notice much of a change in your metabolism as you age.

Symptoms of slow metabolism include fatigue, feeling cold, dry skin, constipation, a slow pulse, low blood pressure, and, of course, weight gain. If you eat a very low-calorie diet, your body will slow its metabolism down in self-defense, holding onto whatever it can in order to survive (your body thinks it is starving). If your diet has resulted in a loss of muscle and an increase in your percentage of body fat, then your metabolism has probably slowed down.

DO YOUR GENES PLAY A ROLE IN METABOLISM?

GENES DO PLAY a role in metabolism. Everyone has a different bone structure and body type. It is not realistic to think that everyone can look like a svelte beach beauty or a muscular body builder. However, given your body type and genetic makeup, you can exercise (with weights and aerobically) to look the best that you possibly can. I must add, despite what you may believe, your genes will not prevent you from achieving your Perfect Weight.

Most experts agree that weight training and aerobic exercise increase metabolism both during and after exercise. They disagree on how long after exercise your metabolism remains increased — that is, how long the "excess post-exercise oxygen consumption" or EPOC lasts. Short-term effects on your metabolism depend mostly on the intensity of the workout, even more so than whether you are exercising aerobically or with weights (although it is far easier to raise your heart rate while exercising aerobically). When you exercise aerobically, focus on burning calories and working your cardiovascular system. Because it takes more calories to exercise, your metabolism speeds up during the activity.

When you are lifting weights or doing other resistance work, you can work out intensely and long enough to raise your heart rate, but most people choose to focus on the activity itself, which not only burns calories, but also increases muscle strength, tone and endurance. This leads to longer-lasting effects on your metabolism. The combination of aerobic activity and weight training will result in a body that has more muscle and less fat, so the end result will be a higher metabolism.

TYPES OF EXERCISE

WALKING

THE SIMPLEST EXERCISE of all, walking, can provide many health benefits: more energy, deeper and more satisfying sleep, stronger leg muscles, less knee pounding than running, lower body fat, a higher metabolic rate, and reduced stress. Daily physical exercise reduces your lifelong risks for heart disease, cancer, stroke, and high blood pressure, and may even slow the aging process.

While 30 to 60 minutes of walking per day is ideal, you can still benefit from increasing your walking by even a small amount. One thing that I highly recommend is to use a pedometer, which counts the steps you actually take during the course of a day and allows you to measure your increases. Aim for a minimum pedometer reading of 10,000 steps every day. One of the best things about walking is that it can be done anywhere; you don't have to make a trip to the gym or take extra time out of your day. Our lifestyles have changed from the past through dependence on vehicles, labor saving devices, sedentary recreation, and a fast-paced lifestyle that leaves little room for dedicated physical activity.

Due to family commitments or other issues, many people have a difficult time setting aside time just for exercising. Walking can be done anywhere. Significant health benefits can come from just 30 minutes of brisk walking on most days. Lunch and breaks are perfect times to get out for some fresh air and a walk around the block. You can also use the stairs instead of the elevator whenever possible, park your car farther away and walk an extra 10 minutes or so to your office, or use the bathroom on a different floor of your office building. When walking, pick up the pace and walk faster!

YOGA

THOSE WHO HAVE never tried yoga are often confused about what it is. Yoga is holding the body in a variety of poses that have been found to be beneficial for (isometric) strength, flexibility, balance, and concentration, and is usually performed in conjunction with breathing exercises and meditation. It may release stress as it is a calming activity. Yoga is extremely effective for the following:

- Increasing flexibility. Yoga has positions that act upon the various joints of the body, including those joints that are rarely exercised. Start by simply taking the time to stretch your arm, neck, and shoulder muscles when sitting in front of the computer. Try a few yoga stretches before bed; your back will thank you.

- Increasing lubrication of the joints, ligaments, and tendons. Likewise, the well-researched yoga positions exercise the different tendons and ligaments of the body. Surprisingly, it has been found that if you start a regular yoga regimen, your body, no matter how rigid you may have felt before, can become remarkably flexible. Why? Seemingly unrelated "non-strenuous" yoga positions act upon certain parts of the body in an interrelated manner, working in harmony to limber us up.

- Massaging of ALL organs of the body. Yoga is perhaps the only form of activity that massages all the internal glands and organs of the body in a thorough manner, including those — such as the prostate — that hardly get externally stimulated during our entire lifetime. Yoga acts in a healthful manner on the various body parts. This stimulation and massage of the organs benefits us by keeping away disease. It can also act as an early warning system for certain diseases or disorders.

- Complete detoxification. By gently stretching muscles and joints as well as massaging the various organs, yoga ensures the optimum blood supply to various parts of the body. This helps flush toxins from every area of the body, which leads to benefits such as delayed aging, restored energy, and a renewed zest for life.

- Excellent toning of the muscles. Muscles that have become flaccid or weak are stimulated repeatedly to shed excess flab and flaccidity. What yoga does is harmonize the mind with the body. Yoga, through meditation, helps the mind work in sync with the body. How often do we find that we are unable to perform our activities properly and in a satisfying manner because the confusions and conflicts in our mind weigh down heavily upon us? Moreover, yoga and meditation effectively counteract stress, which contributes to heart disease (still the number one killer of adult men and women in the U.S.), affecting all parts of our physical, endocrinal, and emotional systems.

The meditative practices through yoga help in achieving an emotional balance by allowing you to temporarily detach from your surroundings, which gives you a remarkable calmness and positive energy that has tremendous benefits on the physical health of the body. These are just some of the tangible benefits that can be achieved through yoga.

It is recommended that you engage in yoga at least twice weekly to benefit from the mind/body connection. If you do not have the time to make it to a yoga class, you can always purchase a yoga DVD and practice yoga in the comfort of your own home first thing in the morning or after the kids go to bed. The Perfect Weight Program includes a yoga DVD, and you may purchase this program at www.bobproctorperfectweight.com.

BENEFITS OF STRENGTH TRAINING

STRENGTH TRAINING USUALLY takes the form of lifting weights, but it can be any activity that provides resistance for the muscles. There are numerous reasons for incorporating strength training into your workout:

- **Increased metabolic rate.** Strength training increases the body's long-term metabolic rate, causing the body to burn more calories throughout the day.
- **Increased and restored bone density.** Inactivity and aging can lead to a decrease in bone density and brittleness. Studies have clearly proven that consistent strength training can increase bone density and prevent osteoporosis.
- **Increased lean muscle mass and muscle strength, power, and endurance.** Everyone can benefit from being stronger. We can work harder, we can play more, we can work out longer, and we can feel more alive.
- **Injury prevention.** Strengthening muscles and joints can prevent a wide variety of sports-related or life-related injuries.
- **Improved balance, flexibility, mobility, and stability.** Stronger and more resilient muscles improve our balance, which means more comfortable living and fewer falls or accidents.

- **Decreased risk of coronary disease.** Participation in a consistent strength-training program has a wide variety of affiliated health benefits, including decreasing cholesterol and lowering blood pressure.

- **Improved rehabilitation and recovery.** One of the best ways to heal many types of injuries is to strengthen muscles surrounding the injured area. The stronger your muscles, the quicker the healing process.

- **Enhanced performance in sports or exercise.** No matter what your favorite sport or physical activity might be, with the proper strength training program, your performance can unquestionably be improved, and in some cases dramatically so.

- **Aging gracefully.** There may be no more important reason to making strength training a consistent part of your life than to ensure you age gracefully. Physical activity keeps you alive and vibrant. Strength training ensures that you are strong enough to participate in aerobic activities, outdoor recreation, sexual activity, and sports. Strong seniors fall down less often, and are less apt to be injured if they do. Their stronger bodies are more resilient, and if they are injured, they heal more quickly.

- **Feeling better and looking better.** Stronger muscles and joints can have a dramatic impact on posture. Lean, toned muscles can also make you feel better about your appearance. This all leads to improved self-esteem and increased self-confidence.

CARDIO TRAINING

CARDIO TRAINING INCLUDES walking, jogging, swimming, or any type of activity that works numerous major muscle groups and gets your heart pumping for the duration of the exercise. You can start by walking, riding a stationary bike, getting on a treadmill or elliptical trainer, using a stair-stepping machine, or doing aerobics. Cardio should be incorporated into your workout regime no fewer than three times weekly.

Once your fitness level begins to improve, you will need to increase the intensity of your cardio training to get past fitness and weight-reduction plateaus. You can do this by incorporating high-intensity intervals into your existing cardio program. If you walk or bike at a fairly consistent pace for 30 minutes, try speeding it up for one minute every few minutes. If you use an aerobics video, you can up the intensity by watching one of the more advanced participants and trying to keep up with them for 30 to 60 seconds at a time. As you become fit, you can try various combinations.

For example, interval training:

- Walk for 10 minutes
- Run for 30 seconds
- Walk for 5 minutes
- Run for 45 seconds
- Walk for 3 minutes
- Run for 1 minute
- Walk for 10 minutes

Once your fitness level increases you can reduce the walking time to three minutes and have one minute of running intervals. (Interval training is one of the most effective methods for fat release as it increases your levels of growth hormone — the hormone responsible for increasing fat breakdown, anti-aging, stimulating the immune system, and increasing muscle repair and growth of all the internal organs except the brain). The key is to constantly challenge your body so you release fat and reduce weight more rapidly. Another benefit of incorporating intervals into your cardio program is that it alleviates boredom. Regular cardio training also helps prevent a variety of diseases, including heart attack, diabetes, high blood pressure, high cholesterol, and obesity. In addition to these health benefits, you can expect to have more energy, higher endurance, and less stress, as well as better sleep, more calories burned, and an easier time achieving your Perfect Weight!

EXERCISE AND EMOTIONS

WITH THE BABY boomers reaching and passing through middle age, more Americans than ever are joining their local gym or health club. The problem is, this isn't enough. You have to actually go. There are as many excuses not to exercise as there are workout wannabes, but here I'd like to concentrate on emotions. If you're like many adults, you feel over-committed, over-scheduled, and over-stressed, and the mere thought of rearranging your life to squeeze in something else feels overwhelming.

So ... don't. That is, don't just rearrange your schedule — change your life. Throughout this book I've emphasized the role the power of the mind plays in your life. By now you know that the first step down the path toward achieving your goals — and your Perfect Weight — is preparing your mind. It's time to stop thinking about what you don't want or think you can't do and replace those thoughts with what you do want and what you can do. This is the perfect time to re-evaluate everything in your life, from how you eat to how you relax. Revisit your priorities now that you've adopted your new, positive mindset, and many of those time and energy commitments you thought would make regular exercise impossible may simply fall by the wayside. You should not feel overwhelmed; you should feel in control.

The good news is that regular exercise can actually help you think positively.

The good news is that regular exercise can actually help you think positively. As with everything else worth achieving, however, that won't happen overnight. When you first begin your new routine, whatever it may be — running, aerobics, swimming, cardio-kickboxing, spinning, circuit training — you'll go through some changes. When you first hit the gym or the trail, you'll feel exhilarated and resolute. And no matter how much exercise you actually manage that first day, when you hit the shower you'll feel pretty darn proud of yourself, and rightly so. But if you aren't used to doing anything physical, after a few hours and especially when you get up the next morning, you'll probably feel exhausted, with aches and pains in muscles that haven't been worked in ages. You may feel that you have barely enough energy to get through the regular parts of your day, let alone exercise. This is temporary! Don't let your body's minor complaints sway your mind's determination to change. No matter how difficult it may be to lace up those running shoes or get up on that stair-step machine, push away those thoughts of "This is too hard" and "I'll never be able to do this." Here's one way to avoid some of that almost-inevitable disillusionment: When you plan your new exercise program, don't design it for your 20-year-old self (unless, of course, you're 20), especially if you've lived a largely sedentary life. Challenge yourself, sure, but don't set goals so unrealistic that you are guaranteed to fail.

Once you make it past the first few days, the first few weeks, and the first few months, you'll notice a strange phenomenon: adding a regular regimen of aerobic activity gives you more energy, not less. That's because your metabolism changes. When you are largely sedentary, your heart pumps oxygen-rich blood to every part of your body at a relatively slow and steady rate. When you exercise enough to raise your heart rate, your blood flows faster, reaching and rejuvenating all your body's cells, and carrying blood to and from your organs—for example, your liver, which (among other things) removes trace toxins and waste elements. Regular exercise also builds up muscle mass, a far more active and efficient metabolizer than, say, love handles and spare tires.

Speaking of energy, don't fall victim to what Dr. Judith Orloff (Positive Energy, Harmony Books) calls "energy vampires." She identifies four types: the constant victim, who recounts every major trauma and minor slight; the charmer, who must be in the spotlight at all times; the drama queen (or king), for whom life is always either incredibly wonderful or a terrible tragedy; and the blamer, whose specialty is making others feel guilty.

These are people who, rather than boosting our spirits and energies, sap it all away, leaving us enervated and distressed. The energy vampires you may meet (and should avoid!) as you introduce your new fitness program are, in Orloff parlance, these: the victim will stop you during your workout to list all the diseases and conditions that keep him or her from being able to do whatever it is you are trying to do; the charmer will teach aerobics or play racquetball with such boundless energy and enthusiasm that you'll feel inadequate and discouraged; the drama queen will get you all excited about a new class and then, when you sign up, tell you that he or she heard that someone died in that class; and finally, the blamer will complain that now that you are exercising, you never spend any time with him or her going to lunch or the movies, or just hanging out. These people are not your friends! Don't let the energy vampires' emotions dampen yours.

Exercising can actually improve your mood, although in the beginning, you may not notice it, or you may even experience the opposite.

Exercising can actually improve your mood, although in the beginning, you may not notice it, or you may even experience the opposite. That's normal. After all, the results of all your exertions are not immediately obvious, and we're not all wired for long-term payoffs. And for some people, particularly those already prone to skin problems, you might have depressing breakouts of acne. The prevention and remedy for that, by the way, are simple: shower as soon as possible after you work up a sweat, preferably with an antibacterial soap.

During and for a while after strenuous exercise, you may feel a significant improvement in your mood. This comes from anandamides, a natural cannabinoid, and endorphins, chemicals released by the pituitary and the hypothalamus glands, which act as natural painkillers and mood boosters. A study done at Duke University Medical Center even showed that engaging in a regular exercise program was as effective in treating mild depression as one of the more popular antidepressants. This "high" can actually help you stick to your routine, as many people become addicted — psychologically, at least.

The difference between try and triumph is just a little umph!

- Marvin Phillips

NOTES

CHAPTER ELEVEN

Getting Support

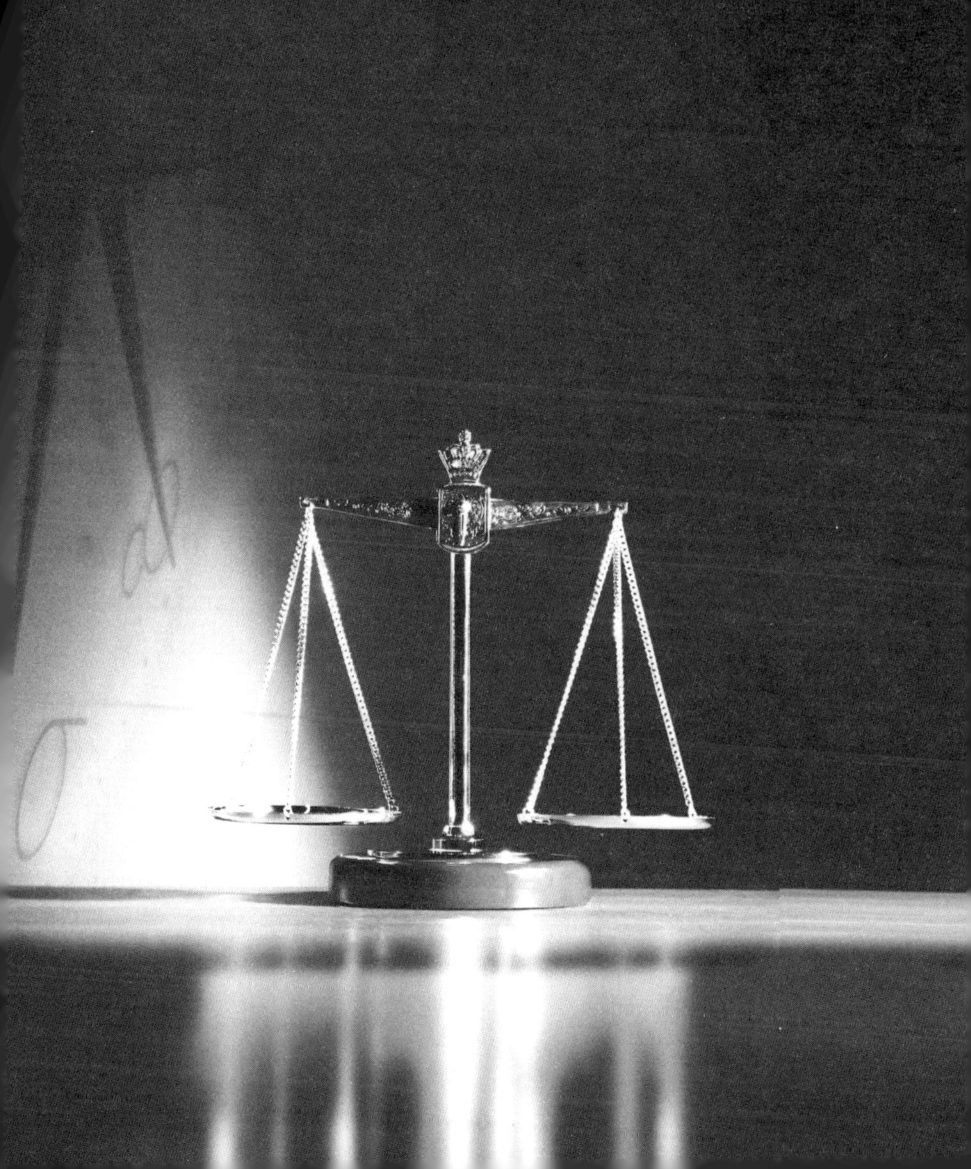

CHAPTER ELEVEN

Getting Support

Obstacles are what we see when we take our eyes off the goal.

– Rita Davenport

It is very hard, if not impossible, to try to make life changes by yourself. None of us lives in a void. We interact with friends, family and coworkers constantly, and these individuals can be a wonderful source of support. Unfortunately, they can also be less than helpful at times and even add to the stress you feel when embarking on a new healthy lifestyle.

I've put together some tips to help you get the most out of your existing support system and some ideas for adding more support from other sources. After all, we all need a little help now and then. When you become truly committed to your new healthy lifestyle, it's perfectly reasonable, and often essential, to ask your loved ones to become key participants along with you.

TIPS FOR GETTING THE BEST SUPPORT FROM FAMILY AND FRIENDS:

1. **Ask for encouragement.** Often we embark on a new exercise regime or weight reduction plan and expect the world to cheer automatically. This doesn't always happen. Let your family and friends know what you're up to, and that you'd like a little boost of encouragement every now and then. Let them know how much you appreciate their support when they help keep you motivated.

2. **Make one area of your house a designated eating zone — and the rest off limits.** This area will probably be the kitchen and/or dining room for most families. Ask everyone's help with no snacking in front of the TV or in their rooms. It's very hard to resist temptation while the person next to you munches buttery popcorn. And don't run out and buy one of those fridges with a TV built in to get around this one!

3. **Put a chart or progress report in plain view for all to see and ask others to celebrate milestones with you (in a non-food celebration).** Your celebration could include going to see a movie (bringing your own snacks) or buying yourself something special. Frequently people have the tendency to keep their weight information private, but if everyone sees your progress, everyone can encourage you — and they may even be inspired to take charge of their own health and eating habits.

4. **Meet with your family or friends and talk about the guidelines of your new program.** Discuss how others can help you meet your goals and pinpoint problem areas before they have a chance to affect your plan. For example, if you frequently have lunch with friends, suggest locations with healthy menu choices.

5. **Clean out the pantry and label one shelf as yours.** Place all your healthy items and snacks on this shelf. When you are tempted to reach for anything in the pantry, your shelf will be right there laden with treats that won't blow your goals. Either ban junk food entirely or insist that it be stored elsewhere.

6. **Learn to share!** Tell others about your successes. When you pass a particular milestone, let others see how enthusiastic and happy you are to be accomplishing your goals. By sharing in your joy, people will see how important this is to you and will therefore be even more likely to support you.

7. **Potluck passion.** Make family get-togethers and dinners healthier by preparing entrees or side dishes that are in keeping with your new eating plan. That way, you will always have something good to eat and you will allow others to have a taste — and maybe even join you.

8. **Plan, plan, plan.** There will often be those in the family who need some convincing that healthy food tastes good. If you have small children or a resistant spouse, be sure to plan meals well in advance so you don't munch from their food choices just because it is quick and easy. Keep track of recipes that you like and that fit with your new

way of eating. Eventually you will have your own great cookbook of healthy and delicious tasting meals so that you don't fall back to your old way of eating.

WHY WON'T THEY HELP?

ANYONE WHO HAS set out on a new healthy lifestyle has encountered a friend or family member who has been less than helpful. It is important to be prepared for the frustrating interference of loved ones who don't approve of or understand your desire to reduce your weight to look and feel better about yourself. Most of us will at some point have someone in our lives who will innocently — or knowingly — try to sabotage our efforts. Usually these types of people have ulterior motives for their desire to keep things as they are, and often it stems from their own insecurities.

Sometimes it all comes down to one ugly four-letter word: fear. Do your friends feel the new, svelte you will move on to things they don't enjoy? Perhaps fellow singletons fear that your social life may improve and you'll be dating instead of socializing with them. Maybe your healthier ways are making your friends feel guilty about their own less-than-perfect eating habits. Or worse, maybe you make them feel better about their own weight issues because they are fat, too, and you may be heavier than they are, so next to you they look and feel thinner.

Many of our social activities revolve around food, dinner with friends, movies with popcorn and soda, happy hour with the gang, or family gatherings. When you change the way you eat, the way you relate to your friends and family (with food) changes, too. To get the "old you" back, some may try to push food on you or try to entice you into joining them in their couch potato existence. A key in preventing or solving this situation is communication. Make it clear from the onset that you're serious about releasing weight and that you need their help to make it happen.

Make it clear from the onset that you're serious about releasing weight and that you need their help to make it happen.

If something like this happens to you, you'll probably find yourself searching for the reasons why — and there isn't an easy answer. Anyone who truly loves you will want what's best for you and your health. If you think you've reached an unhealthy weight and you finally feel ready to change, reducing those excess pounds safely and steadily should become a priority for everyone around you. Eventually most of the people in your life will see that what you're doing is a good thing — even if it does slightly alter your social life or family functions. Do your best to get those around you to not only encourage you, but to also jump on the bandwagon with you toward healthier living. Then everyone benefits.

If you find that you don't get the support you need at home, or if you are new to an area and don't have your normal support system, there are other places to turn. Studies have shown that people who turn to online support are far more likely to succeed in their weight and health goals than those who try to go it alone. Many websites offer forums for those who are going through similar issues to connect and chat. You can start by checking out our website for suggestions (www.bobproctorperfectweight.com). There you'll find that there are always numerous supportive community members ready to talk about healthy eating, share tips on motivation, and discuss whatever else may be on your mind, and you can access this support system any time of the day or night and from anywhere should you feel the need.

Even if you find great support with an online community, sometimes nothing can replace the connection with real people on a personal level. There are also face-to-face support groups you can join if you find the online community a little impersonal.

FOR EXAMPLE:

1. Many community health centers, senior centers, community colleges, and universities offer programs focused on health and well-being. Many will also allow access to medical, nutritional, or fitness specialists for free or a nominal fee.

2. Medical facilities often offer special programs to help with weight issues — especially if you have additional risk factors such as diabetes or high blood pressure. While these wellness programs often cost a bit more, many insurance companies will help with the cost.

3. Join a walking club. If you can't find one in your area, then create one. Studies show that overweight people tend to spend most of their time with other overweight people. Likewise, physically fit people spend their time with other physically fit people. Join a group of physically fit people and you will begin to think like them, which will bring about positive results in both your mind and body!

4. Fitness centers often have nutritionists on staff who can get you involved in their programs and meetings. Don't think you have to spend a lot of money. Often the local YMCA will offer free programs you can join.

5. Be a leader. Why not form your own Perfect Weight club with family, friends, and co-workers? The more people around you who are working toward the same goal, the easier it will be for you!

RELEASING WEIGHT DOESN'T have to mean losing your old friends, and it can even mean making new ones. You could team up with someone and set a date to exercise together. When you make an appointment to work out, you're far more likely to actually show up and do it. Research shows that having a buddy can help you stick to your healthy eating habits, too. A buddy can give you determination when temptation strikes and is only a phone call away. One of my clients and her out-of-town siblings started emailing each other to report the amount of time they spent exercising or walking each day. They had each agreed to commit to at least six hours a week. They nicknamed themselves "skinny minnies," and this has really helped to keep them committed to their goals. This helped them to think twice about sleeping past the alarm in the morning or making an excuse not to go to the gym.

One of the best ways to choose the right person to be your Perfect Weight buddy is to identify your own problem areas. For example, if you tend to snack late at night, find another late-night snacker with whom you can talk on the phone at night rather reaching for that ice cream or chocolate. If the vending machine at work is your weakness, buddy up with a co-worker who also fights the mid-afternoon munchies, and share a walk around the block instead.

The best part about finding another person to team up with is that it is likely your relationship will eventually be about more than eating healthy or working out together. It could be the start of a beautiful friendship that is positive and nurturing.

GET A LIFE OR HEALTH COACH

ONE ALTERNATIVE THAT many people opt for these days is hiring a life coach. Life coaches can help people improve their lives or personal performance in all sorts of areas such as stress management, business, weight reduction, personal relationships, or dozens of other areas. These professionals can help you gain self-knowledge and create more effective goals, as well as help you provide a plan and framework that you will use to go about accomplishing those goals. One of the biggest functions a life coach can provide is assistance with any underlying issues that might be preventing you from succeeding. If you've tried many health regimes in the past and haven't found success, then this is a great option.

TEN WAYS A LIFE OR HEALTH COACH CAN HELP YOU

WHILE LIFE COACHES aren't for everyone, they can provide certain benefits that you can't experience when embarking on the journey alone. Here are 10 reasons a life coach may be right for you:

1. **Motivation.** One of the main benefits of life coaches is that they can offer additional motivation to stick with a consistent program. Life coaches can provide structure and accountability and help you develop a lifestyle that encourages health.

2. **Individualized programs.** If you have any chronic health conditions, injuries, or health goals, life coaches can work with you and your health care provider to plan a safe, efficient program that considers these needs and enables you to reach your goals. Life coaches can also help you determine what goals need to be adjusted depending on those considerations.

3. **Efficiency.** Life coaches help you focus and maintain your purpose. This makes it much easier to stay on target and not waste time starting and stopping your health program.

4. **Improved mental skills.** Once you are able to understand the belief systems that have hindered you in the past, life coaches can encourage new thoughts and affirmations that soon become part of your thought process. This allows you to replace old paradigms with new, positive beliefs about yourself.

5. **Starting points.** If you are an absolute beginner, life coaches can show you tried and true methods to achieve your purpose and vision. They can offer you simple steps to start accomplishing goals that are in line with that purpose and vision.

6. **Break-through plateaus.** Even if you feel you are in relatively good health, life coaches can help you break out of your routine and stretch your boundaries. They will infuse you with new energy, ideas, and passion for life that you may have forgotten over time.

7. **A plan for going it alone.** If you ultimately want to learn all the facets of maintaining your new lifestyle, life coaches can set you on the journey to good health for the rest of your life. Once you understand your own basic motivations and weaknesses, they provide you the tools you will need to take it from there if you choose.

8. **Safe workouts.** Life coaches may also recommend a personal trainer who can watch your form while you exercise and provide objective feedback about your limits and strengths. Exercise isn't a one-size-fits-all approach. There may be certain physical skills you don't have, aren't ready for yet, or that your body doesn't respond to as well. Most of us tend to ignore some of the subtle signals our body provides. We either push through pain or give up too soon. By directing you toward physical activities that you like and that work for you, life coaches can keep your interest high and improve your chances for success.

9. **Convenience.** Many life coaches will accommodate your schedule. This is the number-one reason most people cite

for hiring one. We're all busy, and often gyms and colleges don't offer classes or help when it fits your schedule.

10. **Your Perfect Weight.** As a life coach myself, I specialize in helping people achieve their Perfect Weight. There is a good reason that so many people want a life coach to help. I can keep people on track and help them realize their goals and achieve life-long results. So many of the people I talk with have tried just about everything out there and not met with success in the long-term. Since my approach is first to understand how each person thinks and how that is affecting their outcomes, my clients are able to achieve the long-term success that has eluded them thus far. A healthy lifestyle is not a short-term or one-shot endeavor. It is an ongoing way to live that can bring you tremendous rewards.

FINDING BALANCE

BALANCE MEANS THAT you have a sense that all the parts of your life form a harmonious whole. Balance is different for everyone, and even different for you at various stages of your life. You may work long hours, but if that produces your desired rewards and allows you enough time to enjoy some leisure pursuits while maintaining your health goals, then you're likely to feel balanced and stable.

When you're off-balance, on the other hand, the smallest thing, such as an unexpected deadline, can send you over the edge. Indeed, when things get overwhelming, you lose your balance. This can result in a backslide into old habits — emotional eating, lack of exercise, and a reluctance to try something new. Balance can be a tricky thing to hold onto in your life, as it always seems to be a moving target. The key to balance is to be in control of yourself and your goals, to keep moving in a forward direction, and yet to accept that sometimes you need to take a backward or sideways step to maintain your momentum.

Your sense of balance changes with your life priorities, as the excitement of new goals fades a little and as you become more comfortable with who you are. When you're a young adult, you may be prepared to put a great deal of energy into your work and social life because it may be very important to you to prove yourself, to earn the money you want, and to have fun — while you hardly give your health a second thought. When you reach your 40s and beyond, you may be ready to look past many of your material goals and find you want to spend more time rediscovering yourself and trying out new things. You may also realize that we are given only one body and that failing to take care of it will likely shorten your lifespan, and definitely decrease your quality of life!

I've put together a list of ways you can step back from the chaos and stress of everyday life and enjoy a small moment of balance.

OPPORTUNITIES FOR BALANCE

- Take 10 minutes and envision what you want to achieve. Enjoy the simple act of seeing, hearing, and living your ideal future. Relax and enjoy the moment.

- Understand and remind yourself each day of all you have to be thankful for. A grateful heart allows positive feelings to flow through your body. Take time during each day to list several things you are grateful for, beginning first thing in the morning by saying out loud who and what you are grateful for.
- Balance your own needs and goals with random acts of kindness. Do one thing each day to improve someone else's life. Let someone with only a few groceries go ahead of you, hold a door open, or smile at a stranger.
- Collect wise quotes. Listen and hear the words of those who have been through circumstances like yours and understand their message of hope. I have added quotes in each chapter, so perhaps you can begin with those.
- Read affirmations to yourself every single day. Post them in sight so you can see them easily in times of stress.
- Allow yourself time for reflection. Some days it seems that we go all day without a break. Take a few minutes and allow your mind to reflect on the events of the day.
- Take a few deep breaths and slow down for just a few minutes — in traffic, in line at the store, wherever you are.
- Take a walk. We often spend more time indoors than we realize. Allow yourself a few minutes each day to commune with nature. Notice the change of seasons and allow your heart to soar.
- Be kind to yourself. Forgive any faltering from your plan and keep pushing onward.

Every time you are tempted to react in the same old way, ask if you want to be a prisoner of the past or a pioneer of the future.

- Deepak Chopra

NOTES

CHAPTER TWELVE

Your New Life Begins NOW!

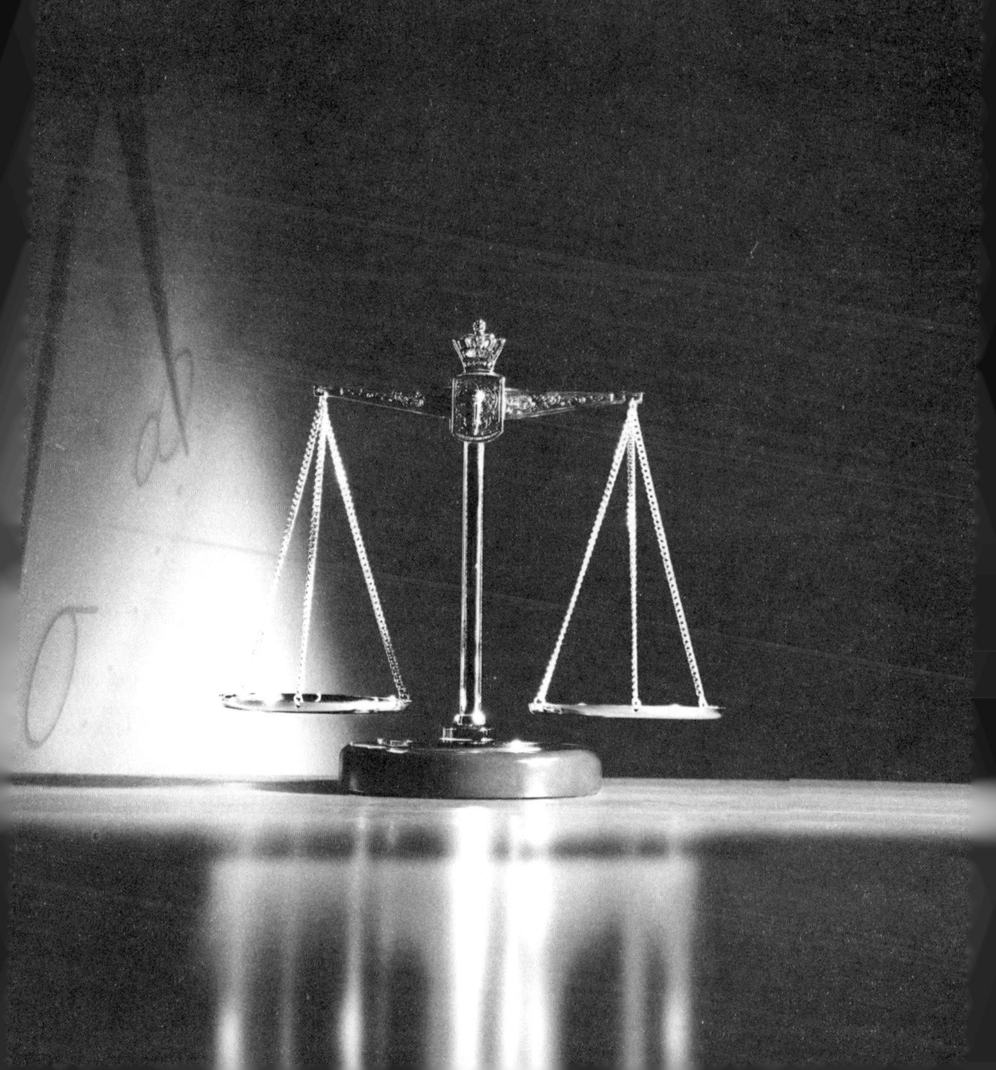

CHAPTER 12
Your New Life Begins NOW!

With the past, I have nothing to do; nor with the future. I live now.

- Ralph Waldo Emerson

As you have read this book, you will have noticed how large a portion of it is spent on preparing your mind to meet your health goals. If you've been involved in weight reduction or fitness programs in the past, you know how hard it is to start again and face the risk of failure. This time is different. Why? Because you believe you can do it now and see the end result in your mind.

We have discussed how obsessed we are as a population with quick fixes and short cuts, and this is not one of them. This is a lifestyle change, not a one-shot proposition. You will not go back to being one of those people who takes good health for granted and continues on the weight-reduction roller coaster ride. The fact that you are searching for answers is the key to finding those solutions.

The purpose of this last chapter is to summarize all that has been covered in this book so that you know where to start and what steps you need to take to ensure that you achieve your goal of attaining your Perfect Weight.

WRITE DOWN YOUR GOAL

WRITE DOWN WHAT your goal is, and see it in your mind's eye. Feel it in your heart and want it with all your might. Find a photo of yourself at your ideal weight, even if you have to cut out a picture from a magazine and paste your smiling face on it. Post it on your fridge, bathroom mirror, inside the cover of this book, your journal, your Perfect Weight Program workbook, or at your desk. When you set your goal, really think about it. As Bob Proctor says, "The goal that is lightly set will be abandoned at the first obstacle." Choose your own goal; others may try to persuade you to follow their vision, but you must pursue your own. You need to own your goal, so be firm about this.

VISUALIZE

Take a look around you. Everything you see was once a thought in someone's mind. Disneyland, the light bulb, the telephone, the car, the airplane — they all started as a small seed of thought in the mind of some brave soul who dared to imagine.

- Bob Proctor

BE SURE TO take the time for yourself each day to visualize your Perfect Weight. As you visualize what you want and create the belief within your sub-conscious mind, the Law of Attraction will assist your efforts by clearing the pathway and allowing you to find those who can help you. This is not to say your path will be without obstacles. If you have struggled with emotional eating in the past, it will occasionally rear its ugly head. As you become more aware of your own triggers, you will be able to abandon this type of eating, along with any "diet victim" excuses you may have used to this point. You have the ability to take control and get what you want. Now use that power to your benefit! As you begin new healthy habits, the daily affirmations you say to yourself will help you through the rough spots.

FOLLOW THE PERFECT WEIGHT NUTRITION PLAN

FOCUS ON HEALTHY eating and become aware of what you put in your mouth and why. Make a copy of the Perfectly Aware Phase and carry it with you. Make several copies: one for your fridge, one for your wallet, and one for your support person or Perfect Weight buddy.

Make sure that you are eating high-quality proteins and fats with each of your four to five daily meals. Choosing vegetables as your primary carbohydrate source will get you to your Perfect Weight more quickly and ensure that you stay there permanently. Reduce and/or eliminate those foods that you have learned will do your body harm; they will impair your digestion. Try to avoid drinking and eating at the same time.

Plan the week's menu in advance and prepare your shopping list to carry with you to the grocery store. Make a point of visiting health food stores and farmers markets where you will find great quality, fresh whole foods. Eat organic whenever possible. By ridding your body of toxins, you will be doing an internal cleansing, and you will soon feel better than you have in years, or even decades! This newfound energy will get you moving off the couch and make you want to start moving and working your muscles. You may find yourself at ballroom dance lessons or wanting to run a marathon. Whatever it is, it will be an excellent boost not only for you but also for those around you. Life is just beginning!

WATER

I NEED TO stress again how important it is to drink plenty of water — specifically alkaline water (refer to section on water for more about alkalinity). Not only is it life giving, it hydrates every cell, allowing your body to function at its highest efficiency. Write down how much water you are currently drinking and what your target is, then write out your plan and commitment to drinking the right amount of water each day.

Set a schedule to get yourself to the ideal level, scheduling it right into your PDA or Day-Timer. If you currently drink two glasses of water a day, increase it gradually. Aim for three tomorrow, then four a few days later, and so on, until you are naturally drinking a minimum of 8 to 10 glasses a day.

The benefits of drinking water are undeniable. You will have more energy, look younger, and feel more vibrant than you have in years. Your skin will radiate its gratitude.

SUPPLEMENTS

DAILY SUPPLEMENTS ARE also important, and some of the more important ones have been outlined for you in Chapter Nine. There may be others that you want to add that you feel will help your particular situation. I've offered only a few of the most important ones, so don't hesitate to add to my list if you feel something additional will benefit you. Remember one thing, though: there is no magic pill, and these supplements should be taken only as a healthy part of your Perfect Weight lifestyle and not as the key ingredient in your nutrition plan. Nothing comes close to the complete nutritional value of fresh food as nature intended.

SUPPORT

I ALSO WANT to reiterate how important it is to get the support you need. Your success is too important to attempt to go it alone. Get everyone you know on your side and rooting for you! If you need to, give your kids a dollar for every time they stop you from putting your hand in their chip bag, ordering French fries, or popping open a cold beer. Hire a life coach and/or a personal trainer — someone trained to assist you in achieving your goals and act as your second conscience. If you have someone to answer to, you'll be more likely to complete a task. Do whatever you feel is necessary to stack the odds in your favor to achieve your ultimate success.

TRACKING

KEEP A WRITTEN log of how you are doing each day. This way you have a record of how far you have come so you can praise yourself for a job well done. Record all that you have eaten (both the healthy and the not so healthy). How much water or other beverages have you consumed? How much activity have you enjoyed? How you are feeling emotionally and physically? How you are sleeping? Did you wake up feeling fantastic and ready to go, or did you want to hide under the covers when the alarm went off? On a scale of 1 to 10, how were your energy levels? What supplements did you take? What positive affirmations did you focus on today? When you begin and then once a month, get out a measuring tape and record your measurements and if you choose to weigh yourself, also only do so once a month. Keep track of how you feel after meals and after eating certain foods. Eliminate those foods that are not causing you to feel well.

REPETITION

REPETITION AND PRACTICE are the keys to learning a new skill. Read this book several times, perhaps a chapter a night. After a couple of weeks, read it again. Review your goal and your motivations to achieve that goal regularly. Never change your actual goal, only the steps required to achieve it if something is not working for you.

In this last chapter, I'd like to get you started on your path to success. The first thing I'm going to ask you to do is take a few minutes and answer some questions about your health and wellness goals. These are designed to make you really think about what you want. They will also uncover some truths about your relationship with food and exercise. Please write your answers in the spaces provided, or in the front of your health journal. This will provide a record of where you started and what your mindset was when you embarked on this journey to your Perfect Weight.

MY HEALTH AND WELLNESS GOALS

1. **How have my feelings about my health and weight changed over the years?**

2. **What's really important to me right now about my health and weight? List as many as you can think of (i.e. getting in shape, reducing my weight, having more energy, etc.).**

3. **Of the areas listed above, which have taken priority for me up to now?**

4. **How has my definition of good health changed over the years? Good health at one time in your life may have meant having the stamina to burn the candle at both ends. Now, good health may mean giving your body rest, and taking care of your mental and emotional well-being through gentle exercise and meditation.**

5. How much time do I want to allocate to my health and well-being? Reaching and maintaining overall good health takes time and effort. Consider whether you want to devote a regular daily time slot to your health goals or if a weekly commitment is better.

6. How do I want to feel when I think about my health? You can translate this desire into a positive affirmation such as, "I feel strong, energetic, and full of vitality every day!"

____

____

____

7. **What do I want for my future health and well-being? Perhaps you want to reduce your weight by twenty pounds or run a marathon, or simply be disease-free and enjoy life.**

____

____

____

____

____

____

THIS SHORT QUIZ will give you a good idea of your starting point. Your body deserves respect and loving care. A great starting point for holistic health (the concept that physical, mental, and emotional health are all connected and have an impact on each other) is getting used to being comfortable in your own skin and changing the way you think and feel about your body. Replace the negative thoughts about your body that pop into your head with positive ones. Succeeding in health and overall well-being usually works best when you focus on what's already working and figure out how to do more of that, or when you enhance what you already have and add great new habits to it.

Hereditary and environmental factors on your health are not always within your full control. No matter what your genetic make up is, however, and no matter what kind of air you have to breathe, you can still actively control and change your diet and the exercise you get. Diet and exercise can make a massive difference in how healthy you are now and will remain throughout your life.

EXERCISE

IF YOU'RE ALREADY fairly healthy, you may just want to take your fitness to the next level. If this is your health goal, then you need to shift into a higher gear and commit to a sustained program that allows you to participate in your chosen exercise for 30 to 60 minutes for at least four out of seven days to achieve a real change in your fitness level. Get out there and do it, and your body will thank you.

Increased fitness gives you more energy on a daily basis, strengthens bones and joints, helps you become more toned, makes you look and feel younger, reduces stress, allows you the ability to join in games with your children, improves your posture, and most importantly, increases your self-esteem. These benefits are all within your grasp through a well-chosen fitness strategy. If you want to achieve all of these benefits, keep the following suggestions in mind:

- Choose a number of different forms of exercise. Start by listing the ones you know you will enjoy. Then list the ones that you'd like to try. Choose at least one from each list.
- Set realistic long-term goals, but always stretch a bit beyond. Begin by checking off the exercises that you know you will do for at least 20 minutes a day.
- Schedule exercise into your PDA with a reminder alarm, or write it on the calendar on your fridge.
- Accept that you need to spend some of your time pursuing your health goals, perhaps at the expense of other activities.
- Choose the form of exercise that works for you as well as inspires and motivates you to keep at it through the days, weeks, and months to come.

EXERCISE AND FITNESS GOALS

FITNESS MEANS DIFFERENT things to different people. Only by examining your preconceived ideas, can you set goals that are in keeping with your overall health goals. Take a few moments and think about these questions.

1. What does "fitness" mean to you? It could mean running a mile in less than five minutes, walking around the block or up a flight of stairs without getting winded, or participating in a triathlon.

2. What environment do you enjoy when you are participating in physical activity? For some this would be the outdoors, for others a gym, and still others prefer team sports. List your preferences.

3. How fit were you when you were young? Were you a star player on the team or a spectator? This will determine your level of understanding of how your body responds to activity and how much you will be able to handle.

4. What environment do you work in and what opportunities does it offer for additional fitness? Does your building have stairs? Do you lift objects frequently? Is there a company sports team you can join? Can you park further away from the entrance?

5. What steps can you take to incorporate fitness into your everyday life? Do you walk to the neighborhood stores and shops? Can you park further away when shopping? Can you walk up and down stairs in your home while on the phone? Think of ways to be active and list them.

____

____

____

____

____

WHETHER YOUR EXERCISE of choice is strapping on a pedometer and setting off on a walk or practicing yoga, I would encourage you to occasionally change your routine in order to keep things interesting. Don't forget that physical activity has a direct and positive impact on your mental well-being. It can also be very helpful in managing your emotions.

Do you feel comfortable expressing your emotions, or do you bottle things up only to find they explode at just the wrong moment? Do you notice what your emotions are all the time, or do you find you sometimes feel upset but can't really put your finger on why? Often when our physical well-being is out of sync, our emotions are as well. This can result in anger, emotional tears, and even panic. These emotions have a physical effect on the body that can be released through regular, healthy exercise. Exercise gives your mind a chance to work through any emotional issues, and it also releases endorphins, a natural chemical released by the pituitary gland that spreads a feeling of calm and happiness through the body.

Recall times when you've experienced various emotions and describe what the physical feeling is for you. Perhaps "joy" or "pride" brings on a warm sensation to the back of your throat. Or thinking of the word "motivation" causes a pleasant tension in your abdomen. Notice the similarities and differences between each positive emotion. Now think about the negative emotions that you experience. Maybe "anger" causes your shoulders to tense while "lonely" gives you an empty feeling in your stomach.

A positive thought is not just an idea; it has a positive physical effect and regular exercise can increase that effect.

A positive thought is not just an idea; it has a positive physical effect. Regular exercise can increase that effect. Armed with this awareness, you can now watch yourself as you go about your day and notice your feelings. When someone cuts you off in traffic, how do you feel? Angry? Frustrated? Rejected? You might be surprised at the real emotion behind the trigger and that it can change depending on the mood you're in to begin with. By maintaining a positive outlook, it is less likely that a negative event will ruin your day or steer you off course from achieving your Perfect Weight goal.

You can make a big impact on your emotional well-being by simply noticing the things that make you feel good and going out of your way to make them part of your life. Those mornings when you wake up full of enthusiasm for no particular reason don't come out of thin air. Your mind takes what you give it, and if you're supplying positive thoughts while feeding your body healthy food and exercising regularly, then of course you will wake up feeling great on most days! That is a welcome and gratifying way to start your day.

Eventual success will depend on your level of mental resilience and how quickly you can bounce back from setbacks. If you feel that you're wobbling on the edge, about to slide into old habits due to external pressures and feeling out of control, you're not alone. Many people who seem to be very healthy and fit have at some time or another suffered from weight gain and couch potato syndrome. Recently a friend of mine went hiking in the snow. The next day her thighs were extremely sore, but her husband wanted to go hiking again. Even though it was snowing hard, they headed out anyway. Before long she started complaining about how sore her legs were and swearing that she didn't think she could continue. All she could think of was how good it would feel to get back home and put her feet up. Her husband was the support she needed that day. He kept her focused on the moment, reminded her how toned her legs were going to be, and described the nice bath she could take when she was finished the hike. She persisted through the discomfort. She did reward herself with a hot bubble bath later that night, but what felt even better was her feeling of accomplishment!

Developing mental resilience begins with some basic strategies that can help you grow stronger:

- Talk to people who can help you when you experience setbacks, like life coaches.
- Sometimes you simply need a friend who can be there for you. You don't get an award for bravery for going it alone. Enlist the advice of a doctor or trained counselor if volatile emotions become persistent and overwhelming.
- Keep focused on your priorities. You may need to practice saying "no" from time to time. When you feel less mentally resilient, you may try to please people more, or go in the other direction and get angry at the demands they place on you. Knowing your goals and reminding yourself of them often can be the sanity check you require to assert your needs.
- Schedule a regular activity that builds your mental and emotional muscles. Take note of activities that leave you with a sense of peace and perspective and give them priority in your life. This may mean going to a particular place where you like to meditate, or engaging in an active sport you enjoy.
- Take the performance pressure off yourself. You are the most important person in your world; however, you must realize that everyone around you is far too caught up in his or her own anxieties and issues to notice yours. Remember that you don't have to be perfect; be content with being good enough. Be kind to yourself.

ALL OR NOTHING

ONE OF THE biggest problems I've seen with people who are excited and start a new healthy eating program is that they have an "all-or-nothing" attitude. They want to get slim overnight and quickly become frustrated. When you want to reduce a significant amount of weight, it's easy to fall into all-or-nothing thinking. This kind of thinking can create a certain air of desperation, which may cause you to rationalize it with arguments similar to these:

- You have to follow a super-strict diet to succeed.
- If you fall off the wagon and eat junk for a day or two, you've blown it altogether so you may as well give up.

This line of thinking can be very detrimental to your weight reduction efforts, but it's all too easy a trap to fall into. Since how you think about your program is the most important area, I've compiled a short list of helpful hints to get your thoughts back on track if you find yourself taking one step forward and three steps back.

HELPFUL HINT #1: LOOSEN UP.

THE FIRST WAY to avoid all-or-nothing thinking is to shake the idea that you must follow an extremely restrictive diet to reduce your weight. The fact is, most people who successfully manage their weight don't diet at all. They make healthy, permanent lifestyle changes such as cutting back on overall calories, practicing portion control, making better food choices, finding a hobby that gets them outdoors, and reigning in emotional eating. Successful weight reduction focuses on weight management, not just weight reduction.

HELPFUL HINT #2: HAVE A BITE OR TWO!

SEVERELY LIMITING YOUR food intake or completely cutting out your favorite foods sets you up to binge. Temptation becomes much less powerful when you can have just a taste of something off limits now and again instead of telling yourself it's off limits for good. This can be difficult at first, but you will become accustomed to satisfying your cravings with smaller amounts of these tempting foods and learn to enjoy them on occasion in small quantities with just a bite or two!

HELPFUL HINT #3: REMOVE THE WORD "DIET" FROM YOUR VOCABULARY!

MANY PEOPLE GO on and off diets after every holiday season. They say, "I'll start my diet in the New Year," only to be off it by the next weekend. You never hear anyone say, "I'll start my new way of life Monday," but that's exactly what we need to do. An effective program or lifestyle isn't just to get you ready for bikini season; it's to keep you ready for life.

HELPFUL HINT #4: FORGIVE YOURSELF.

LET'S SAY YOU'VE decided to give Helpful Hint #2 a try and allow yourself your favorite treat, chocolate chip cookies. But you don't stop at a couple ... you eat half the package. Then, for breakfast tomorrow morning ... you polish off the other half. Have you completely blown it again? Does that mean it's time to give up altogether? Do you think, "Maybe I'm just not cut out for this" and go back to your old eating habits? Not allowing yourself to make mistakes is the worst error you can make.

Think about this: all-or-nothing thinking is a way to let you off the hook. It's an escape route "Oh, now I've screwed up. Glad I don't have to bother anymore." There's an old saying that goes, "No matter how far along you are down the wrong path, it's never too late to turn back." So don't think that just because you made a bad choice today you can't start over tomorrow, or even later that same day! It sounds like a cliché, but every day, actually every moment, truly is a new beginning. You can't erase last night's binge, but you can aim for a much healthier today!

HELPFUL HINT #5: CELEBRATE SMALL VICTORIES.

PRAISE YOURSELF FOR the small challenges you surmount; you won't give up so easily if you do. Yes, choosing fish instead of beef is a victory. Doing an exercise video on Friday is a triumph, even if it's the first day you've exercised this week. Take it easy on yourself as you're learning how to be a new, improved, healthier you. Just don't do it with your feet up!

No matter what health or fitness program you choose, it will be an adjustment for your life. You may not always get it right the first time. Quite often it's the process of making adjustments that tells you exactly what and how much you need of certain things in your life. Think hard about whether you have too much or too little of something in your life. In fact, you may have good reasons why you made the balance tip in a certain direction over time. Have you become bored with your eating regime or your exercise routine? Spice it up and beware of boredom! Be honest about what you want and don't want in your life. How important this goal of good health is will shift over time, and that's normal. As long as you are paying attention to your body and living a healthy lifestyle, it's okay to cut back to a couple of times per week at the gym. You don't have to maintain the same regime that helped you get in shape once you're there. Just be sure it doesn't fall by the wayside altogether.

ARE YOU ABLE AND ARE YOU WILLING?

LET'S TAKE THESE questions one at a time. Am I able? ... are you able to receive, in your physical world, anything you seriously want? It was Napoleon Hill who said that you will not seriously want something that you are not capable of achieving.

The second question you must answer is this: "Am I willing?" Are you willing to pay the price that must be paid, realizing that there is no such thing as something for nothing and that nature abhors a vacuum? You must create a space for the good that you desire. Everyone's life is full at all times. The question you must ask yourself is, "What is it full of?" Before you can do something else, you must stop whatever it is that you're doing and create a space for what you desire.

Are you willing and able to ...
Make an investment in yourself?
Go where you have to go? Do what you have to do?
Change what you have to change?
Let go of what has to go? Study what must be studied?
Take direction when it is required?
Continue in the face of failure?
Make a 100% commitment to yourself that you will reach your Perfect Weight?

If your answer is yes, a resounding, "YES – I AM WILLING," *you are already on your way to being at your Perfect Weight. The material changes must, by natural law, follow.*

- Bob Proctor

BY FOLLOWING THE methods set forth in this book, you will not only achieve your Perfect Weight, but you will also gain a new lifestyle that will provide you with a healthy and energetic body and mind. The lessons discussed in the first several chapters can be applied to so many areas of your life and will help you with achieving any goal that you desire. I encourage you to check out our website at www.bobproctorperfectweight.com to download some healthy recipes and articles. I wish each of you much success with your journey of achieving your Perfect Weight and living the healthiest, happiest life possible.

Bob Proctor

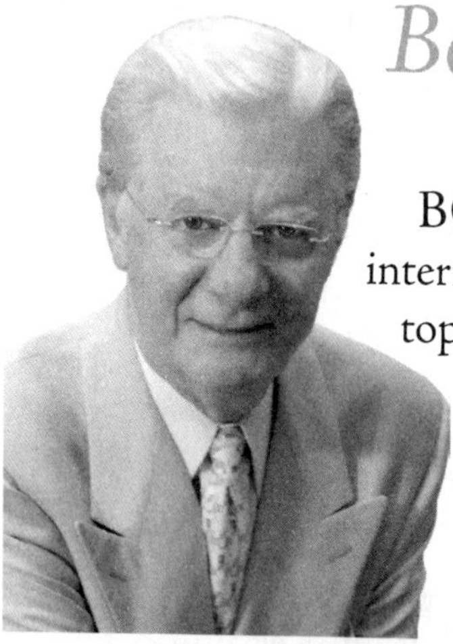

BOB PROCTOR IS an internationally renowned speaker on the topic of achieving your dreams. For the last 40 years he has taught people how to uncover and capitalize on the image of perfection that lies within every person. This new awareness leads to the expression of your hidden abilities to be more, do more and have more in every area of life.

Through his own personal struggle and then triumph, Bob understands the cyclical trap which can easily convince you that your efforts are wasted. He shares the basis behind these beliefs and how to overcome them, leading you to freedom.

Bob knows that each and every person has the power to change their life in positive ways; listen to what he says and you will be convinced. By removing the mystery of how we think and why achieving our Perfect Weight is such an enormous challenge, he clears the path for you to achieve more than you ever thought possible. You are going to love this new program.

Over the last four decades, millions have heard Bob's revolutionary message of empowerment and inner strength that is the birthright of every person. He now travels the globe, teaching thousands of people how to believe in and act upon the greatness of their own minds. Bob is very enthused about teaming up with Melonie Dodaro and the power they have created in this program, he is one of Melonie's biggest fans.

Melonie Dodaro

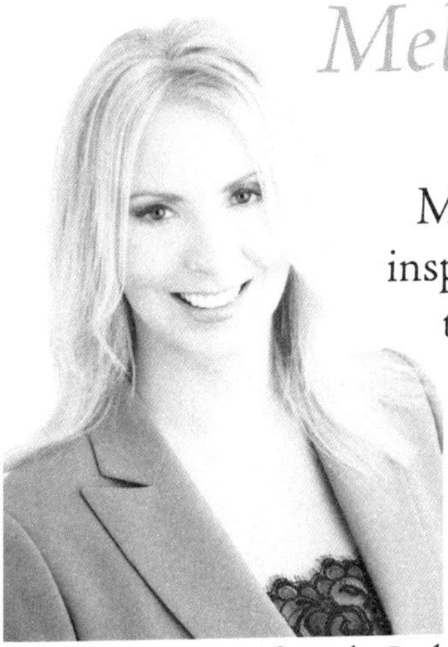

MELONIE DODARO WAS inspired to write this book by the teachings of the mind by Bob Proctor. Having studied with many of the teachers from "The Secret" she was prompted to achieve her goal of helping people reach their weight reduction objectives by aligning herself with Bob Proctor to create the Perfect Weight Program. Her work with these inspirational and talented life coaches motivated her to create the perfect program for weight reduction success by introducing the missing ingredient, the mind.

Melonie is an expert in this industry having gained vast knowledge and experience helping thousands of clients during her 10 successful years in the weight loss industry as an owner of several weight loss centers. She has developed a winning program for people from all walks of life to overcome their battle with the bulge. Her words will inspire you to find the path to your Perfect Weight. As you work towards that significant goal you will learn the life lessons the world's most successful people already have put into practice in their everyday lives. Follow the simple path Melonie has laid out for you and you will be the weight you want to be and create everything in your life you ever dreamed of.